Handbook of Canine & Feline Urinalysis

by
Carl A. Osborne, DVM PhD*
and
Jerry B. Stevens, DVM, PhD§

* Professor and Chairman,
  Department of Small Animal Clinical Sciences

§ Professor,
  Department of Veterinary Pathobiology
  College of Veterinary Medicine,
  University of Minnesota,
  St. Paul, MN 55108

RALSTON PURINA COMPANY: Checkerboard Square, Saint Louis, Missouri 63188
©Copyright 1981 by Ralston Purina Company.
Copyright under the International Copyright Union
All rights reserved.
This book is protected by copyright.
Made in the United States of America.

Photographs reproduced by permission.

Library of Congress catalog number: 81-52449
First printing, 1981

Preface

"*Wisdom is the prime thing. Acquire wisdom, and with all that you acquire, acquire understanding.*"

Proverbs 4:7.

Macroscopic and microscopic examination of urine can provide a wealth of diagnostic and prognostic information, and may be used as an index of therapeutic response. Urinalysis is one of the most important diagnostic tools available to veterinarians. Every veterinarian in clinical practice should do all possible to master laboratory techniques and interpretation of analysis of this golden liquid.

The reliability of results of urinalysis are significantly influenced by conceptual understanding of physiologic processes governing urine formation, storage, and elimination, urine collection techniques, methods of urine preservation, and laboratory methods. Proper perspective in evaluation of results is also dependent on conceptual understanding of the difference between observations and interpretations of observations. We have endeavored to incorporate these principles throughout this handbook of urinalysis. Our goal has been to provide information in a readily comprehendible and easy-to-find outline form.

Time and experience have polished the thought that "A FACT MERELY MARKS THE POINT WHERE WE HAVE AGREED TO LET INVESTIGATION CEASE." It is undoubtedly a fact, however, that not all of our colleagues will agree with the observations and interpretations we have advanced herein. We apologize for our shortcomings, and invite those who would help us to correct them to bring them to our attention. One way to advance truth is by vigorous and open interaction of opposing opinions.

C.A.O.
J.B.S.

Table of Contents

URINALYSIS

VETERINARY HOSPITALS-UNIVERSITY OF MINNESOTA

Lab No. _____

CLINICIAN	STUDENT-ASSISTANT	DATE

☐ Routine Urinalysis   Other _____

	TIME COLLECTED	TIME ANALYZED

Problem

Clinician's Comments

Collection Technique
☐ By Owner   ☐ Manual Compression   ☐ Cystocentesis
☐ Micturition   ☐ Catheterization   ☐ Table Top, Cage, Floor

☐ Refrigerated   ☐ Preservative added _____

CASE NO.
OWNER
ADDRESS
CITY, STATE

ANIMAL
SPECIES
BREED
AGE
SEX
NAME/TAG NO.

TOTAL FEE: _____

Color	Micro Exam ☐ 5ml Other _____ ml		
Odor	RBC	/HPF	WBC /HPF
Turbidity	CASTS	Hyaline/LPF	
Specific Gravity		Granular/LPF	
pH		Other/LPF	
Glucose (glucose oxidase)	Epithelial Cells OCC FEW MOD MANY/HPF		
Glucose (copper reduction)	Epithelial Cells Type		
Ketones	Fat Droplets OCC FEW MOD MANY/HPF		
Bilirubin	Sperm OCC FEW MOD MANY/HPF		
Occ Bd; Hb; Myoglb.	Bacteria FEW MANY	Bacteria Shape	
Protein (dipstick)	Crystals OCC FEW MOD MANY/HPF		
Protein (SSA)	Crystals Type		

24 hr. Urine Protein	gm/24 hrs.	3.00
Total Urine Vol _____ ml ☐ 24 hr___ml		
Urobilinogen Screen		1.00
Urobilinogen Quantitative	Erl. U.	5.00
Osmolality	mOsm.	5.00
Comments:		

TECHNOLOGIST _____ DATE _____

Fig. 1. Laboratory form for recording the results for a routine urinalysis.

Chapter 1. Definition of Terms and Concepts

Table 1
Normal Findings—Fresh Canine and Feline Urine

COMPONENT	ADULT DOG	ADULT CAT
Color	Yellow	Yellow
Turbidity	Clear	Clear
Specific gravity:		
minimum	1.001	1.001
maximum	1.065+	1.080+
typical range	1.015–1.045	1.035–1.060
Volume (ml/lb body wt./day)	±12 to 20*	±8 to 10*
Osmolality:		
minimum	50	50
maximum	±2,400	±3,000
typical range	500–1,200	?
pH	4.5–8.5	4.5–8.5
Glucose	Negative	Negative
Ketones	Negative	Negative
Bilirubin	Trace to 1+**	Negative
Occult Blood	Negative	Negative
Protein	Trace**	Negative
RBC/HPF	0–5(?)	0–5(?)
WBC/HPF	0–5(?)	0–5(?)
Casts/LPF	Occasional hyaline	Occasional hyaline
Epithelial/HPF	Occasional	Occasional
Fat Droplets/HPF	Uncommon	Common
Bacteria/HPF	Negative	Negative
Crystals/HPF	Variable	Variable

*Guesstimates only
**In highly concentrated urine.

Definition of Terms and Concepts

I. THE COMPLETE ROUTINE URINALYSIS

In our hospital, a complete routine urinalysis consists of evaluation of several physical and chemical properties of urine, estimation of its solute concentration, and microscopic examination of urine sediment (Figure 1, Table 1). We recommend that all of these tests be performed because they aid in semiquantitation and localization of abnormal findings, and refinement of problems. For example, interpretation of the results of chemical tests (and sediment examination) is aided by knowledge of urine specific gravity (an indirect index of the volume of urine produced).

The value of microscopic examination of the urine sediment in the interpretation of urinalyses is comparable to microscopic examination of blood smears in the interpretation of hemograms. Meaningful interpretation of physical (color, turbidity) and chemical (protein, occult blood, pH) test results of routine urinalyses are dependent on knowledge of the composition of urine sediment. For example, a moderate degree of proteinuria in absence of significant numbers of red cells and white cells usually indicates proteinuria of glomerular origin. A moderate degree of proteinuria associated with hematuria and pyuria, however, indicates an inflammatory response somewhere along the urinary and/or genital tracts.

II. QUALITATIVE, SEMIQUANTITATIVE, AND QUANTITATIVE URINALYSES

A. Because the concentration of solutes, cells, *etc.*, varies with the quantity of water being excreted at a particular time, urine samples collected without regard to rate of urine formation (*i.e.*, number of milliliters *per* unit of time) are only suitable for qualitative and semiquantitative determinations.

1. Daily variation in urine volume and composition influenced by eating, drinking, metabolism, and various diseases must be considered when interpreting test results.

2. Pseudo-precision implied by urine specific gravity values conventionally measured in thousandths of a unit (*i.e.*, 1.001 to 1.060+) and solutes (glucose, protein, *etc.*) listed as mg/100 ml should not be over-interpreted.

3. Randomly collected urine samples are usually suitable for diagnostic screening; however, measurement of substances in urine obtained during timed intervals may be subsequently required to clarify the significance of questionable results.

B. Collection of urine specimens during a specified time period is required for quantitative determination of excretion rates of endogenous and/or exogenous substances.

1. For quantitation of endogenous substances (protein, hormones, electrolytes, *etc.*), 24-hour urine collections are usually preferred since they eliminate diurnal variations in urine excretion. To verify the existence and/or determine the magnitude of polyuria, 24-hour urine collections may also be used.

a. A metabolism cage is frequently used to collect all urine formed during a 24-hour interval. In some situations, a shorter time interval may be used; values may be prorated to a 24-hour interval. For best results, the urinary bladder should be emptied and the urine discarded at the beginning of the collection period. It should be emptied again at the end of the procedure, but the urine should be included in the calculation.

b. When possible, the patient should be allowed to acclimate to the environment of the metabolism unit for a day or so before the beginning of the study.

c. Reproducible 24-hour collections are notoriously difficult to obtain. The best data are usually obtained by measuring and comparing urine output (and water intake) for each of two or three days.

d. Quantitation of substances in urine may be obtained by measuring the quantity in a representative aliquot of the 24-hour sample, and correcting this value for the 24-hour volume.

2. For quantitation of exogenous substances, exogenous creatinine clearance, urinary excretion of phenolsulfonphthalein dye, *etc.*, shorter time intervals are commonly used.

a. Inability of most animals to co-operate in timing of voiding usually requires use of urinary catheters.

b. Swan Ganz flow-directed balloon catheters are recommended for timed urine collections (refer to Chapter 4, Collection Techniques, for further information).

III. OVERVIEW OF URINE FORMATION AND ELIMINATION

The urinary system plays a major role in maintaining homeostasis by eliminating metabolic waste products from the body. In addition, the kidneys produce and degrade a variety of hormones. A conceptual understanding of renal function is an essential prerequisite for determination of optimum times of urine collection for analysis of specific components, and for interpretation of results.

Formation of urine by the kidneys results from three basic processes:

1. Glomerular filtration.
2. Tubular reabsorption.
3. Tubular secretion.

These mechanisms are modified by several hormones of non-renal origin including antidiuretic hormone, aldosterone, parathormone, thyrocalcitonin, prohormone (vitamin) D, prostaglandins, calcitonin, and thyroxine.

It was well-established that formation of glomerular filtrate from plasma is a major function of glomeruli. Glomerular filtration is a passive process for the kidneys, deriving its energy from pressure generated by contraction of the left ventricle and the elasticity of vascular walls. Factors which influence the quantity and quality of glomerular filtrate include (Table 2):

1. Hydrostatic pressure.
2. Volume of blood in glomerular capillaries.
3. Colloidal osmotic pressure of blood in glomerular capillaries.

Table 2

Classification of Altered Glomerular Filtration and Azotemia

CAUSE	CLASSIFICATION OF AZOTEMIA
Decreased blood volume	Prerenal
Decreased blood pressure	Prerenal
Decreased colloidal osmotic pressure	Prerenal
Decreased number of patent vessels	Primary renal
Decreased glomerular permeability	Primary renal
Increased renal interstitial pressure	Primary renal
Increased intratubular pressure	Primary renal (tubular obstruction)
Increased intratubular pressure	Postrenal (obstruction of ureters, bladder, urethra)

4. The number of patent renal vessels and glomerular capillaries.
5. The permeability of glomerular capillaries.
6. Renal interstitial pressure.
7. Renal intratubular pressure.

Hydrostatic pressure is the major force which favors glomerular filtration. Forces which oppose glomerular filtration include colloidal osmotic pressure (which arises primarily from non-filtered protein molecules in glomerular capillary plasma), renal intratubular pressure, and the selective permeability of glomerular capillary walls. Renal interstitial pressure is negligible under normal conditions, but may oppose glomerular filtration if it becomes abnormally elevated.

The glomerulus functions as a sieve which increasingly restricts passage of macromolecules of increasing diameter and molecular weight. Although the ability of many substances to traverse glomerular capillary walls is related to their molecular weight, the shape or configuration of molecules, as well as their electrical charge, also are important variables that influence the degree to which some substances are filtered. Since cells, most proteins, and most lipoproteins are too large to pass through glomerular capillary walls, they are retained within the vascular compartment and are not present in glomerular filtrate in significant quantities. The negative charge of proteins also restricts their filtration since glomerular capillary walls have a negative charge. Most substances in glomerular filtrate of mammals have a molecular weight of less than 68,000 (Table 3). Thus glomerular filtrate is qualitatively similar to plasma with respect to the concentration of electrolytes and small molecular weight substances.

Table 3
Comparison of Molecular Weights of Substances Included in, and Excluded from, Glomerular Filtrate

SUBSTANCE	MOLECULAR WEIGHT	PRESENCE IN GLOMERULAR FILTRATE
Water	18	+
Urea	60	+
Creatinine	113	+
Glucose	180	+
Lysozyme	14,000	+
Myoglobin	17,000	+
Bence Jones Monomers	22,000	+
Bence Jones Dimers	44,000	+
Amylase	50,000	+
Hemoglobin*	68,000	±
Albumin	69,000	±
Immunoglobulin-G	160,000	−
Immunoglobulin-A (Dimer)	300,000	−
Fibrinogen	400,000	−
Alpha-2-Macroglobulin	840,000	−
Immunoglobulin-M	900,000	−

*Probably excreted as a dimer with a molecular weight of approximately 32,000.

The common denominator of substances which appear in glomerular filtrate is not their potential value to the body, but rather their size, shape, and electrical charge. In order for the kidneys to regulate body fluid, electrolyte and acid-base balance, it is essential that both beneficial and worthless metabolites with similar characteristics be subjected to potential loss in urine.

Some filtered substances (*i.e.*, allantoin and creatinine) cannot be reutilized by the body and are not reabsorbed by the tubules. Other filtered substances (*i.e.*, amino acids, vitamins, glucose) are essential for body homeostasis, and are almost completely reabsorbed by the tubules. The body's requirement for water, electrolytes and other filtered substances is variable, being dependent upon intake, metabolism and loss from nonrenal routes. Nephrons regulate conservation and excretion of these substances by selective partial tubular reabsorption and tubular secretion. The ability of the kidneys to help maintain water balance, despite wide variation in water intake, is dependent on the complex interaction of factors influencing circulating concentrations of several hormones (antidiuretic hormone, aldosterone, *etc.*) and factors influencing the renal medullary countercurrent system. Thus as glomerular filtrate passes through the tubules, it loses its original identity. The overall effect of these tubular functions is to balance the loss and gain of metabolites and water initially present in glomerular filtrate according to body need.

The kidneys are involved in regulation of erythropoiesis by production of erythropoietin, of calcium homeostasis by metabolizing vitamin (prohormone) D to its most metabolically active form, and of fluid and electrolyte balance by formation of renin and prostaglandins. The kidneys also degrade hormones, including parathormone, insulin and thyrotropic hormone.

The hydrodynamics associated with collection and unidirectional transport of urine from the renal pelvis to the bladder and its subsequent elimination by the process of micturition are also essential for body homeostasis. Urine that accumulates in the renal pelvis initiates peristaltic movement of pelvic and then ureteral smooth muscle. As a result, elongated boluses of urine are propelled through the ureteral lumen to the urinary bladder. Anatomic ureterovesical sphincters are not present; however, the oblique course of the ureters through the bladder wall at the trigone forms a flap valve that normally prevents retrograde flow of urine from the bladder. Ureterovesical valves protect the kidneys from abnormal retrograde pressure, and from contamination with infected bladder urine.

Micturition consists of the storage of urine in the urinary bladder, and its periodic complete elimination through the urethra. Micturition is fundamentally a reflex facilitated and inhibited by higher brain centers and, like defecation, is subject to voluntary initiation and inhibition.

IV. TERMS AND CONCEPTS RELATED TO URINE CONCENTRATION AND DILUTION

A. **BARURIA:** Urine of high specific gravity and high osmolality.

B. **CONCENTRATION OF URINE:** Tubular modification of glomerular filtrate so that more water is removed than solute. The specific gravity of glomerular filtrate is approximately 1.008 to 1.012, while the osmolality is approximately 300 mOsm/liter. Concentrated urine has a higher specific gravity and higher osmolality than glomerular filtrate.

C. **DILUTION OF URINE:** Tubular modification of glomerular filtrate so that more solute is removed than water. Dilute urine has a lower specific gravity and lower osmolality than glomerular filtrate.

D. **HYPERSTHENURIA:** Urine of high specific gravity and high osmolality.

E. **ISOSTHENURIA:** Urine with a specific gravity and osmolality similar to that of plasma and glomerular filtrate.

Impaired ability to concentrate or dilute glomerular filtrate according to body need is sometimes called "fixed specific gravity."

F. **OSMOLALITY:** The property of a solution which is dependent on the concentration of osmotically active particles in solution. For osmolality the unit of solvent measurement is mass (kilograms), and therefore osmolality is expressed as mOsm/kg of solution. For osmolarity the unit of solvent measure is volume (liter), and therefore osmolarity is expressed as mOsm/L of solution.

G. **SPECIFIC GRAVITY:** Urine specific gravity is a measurement of the density of urine compared to pure water. Urine specific gravity is the ratio of the weight of urine to the weight of an equal volume of water, both measured at the same temperature. Because specific gravity is a ratio, it is not followed by a unit of measurement.

V. TERMS AND CONCEPTS RELATED TO RENAL DISEASE, RENAL FAILURE, AND UREMIA

A. Confusion caused by use of the terms azotemia, renal disease, renal failure, and uremia as synonyms may result in misdiagnosis and formulation of inappropriate, and even contraindicated therapy.

B. DEFINITIONS

1. AZOTEMIA

    a. Azotemia is defined as the presence of abnormal concentrations of urea, creatinine and other nonprotein nitrogenous substances in blood, plasma, or serum.

    b. Azotemia is a laboratory finding and may or may not be caused by generalized lesions of the renal parenchyma.

    c. Nonrenal causes of azotemia (prerenal and postrenal) associated with decreased glomerular filtration rate include decreased blood volume, decreased blood pressure, decreased colloidal osmotic pressure, and obstruction of both ureters, the bladder or urethra (*see* Table 2).

2. RENAL FAILURE

    a. Failure is defined as inability to perform.

    b. The kidneys perform multiple functions in maintaining homeostasis, including elimination of waste products of metabolism from the body, synthesis of a variety of hormones, and degradation of a variety of hormones.

c. Failure to perform these functions may not be an "all or none" phenomenon. For example, in slowly progressive renal diseases, failure of the ability to concentrate or dilute urine according to body needs typically precedes failure to eliminate waste products of metabolism. In turn, laboratory detection of impaired ability to maintain electrolyte and nonelectrolyte solute balance typically precedes onset of polysystemic clinical signs caused by renal dysfunction. In some situations renal disease may precede renal failure, and likewise, renal failure may precede uremia. In many instances renal disease does not progress to a state of renal failure.

d. The concept that adequate renal function is not synonymous with total renal function is of importance in:
   (1) Understanding the difference between renal disease and renal failure.
   (2) Formulating meaningful prognoses.
   (3) Formulating specific, supportive and symptomatic therapy.

3. UREMIA

a. Uremia is defined as the presence of abnormal quantities of urine constituents in blood caused by primary generalized renal disease and the polysytemic toxic syndrome which occurs as a result of abnormal renal function.

b. Although uremia is always accompanied by azotemia and renal failure, azotemia and renal failure may or may not be associated with uremia.

C. RENAL DISEASE

1. Renal disease indicates the presence of renal lesions of any size, distribution (focal or generalized), or cause (anomalies, infection, endogenous or exogenous toxins, obstruction to urine outflow, neoplasms, ischemia, immune disorders, hypercalcemia, trauma) in one or both kidneys. The specific cause of renal disease(s) may or may not be known; however, quantitative information about renal function (or dysfunction) is not defined.

2. Renal disease cannot be used synonymously with renal failure and uremia because of the tremendous reserve capacity of the kidneys.

a. Depending on the quantity of renal parenchyma affected and the severity and duration of the lesions, renal diseases may or may not cause renal failure and uremia.

b. Impairment of urine concentrating and diluting capacity of canine kidneys cannot be detected by evaluation of urine specific gravity or urine osmolality until approximately two-thirds of the total renal parenchyma is surgically extirpated.

c. Although the serum concentrations of urea nitrogen and creatinine vary inversely with glomerular filtration rate, approximately three-fourths of the nephrons of both kidneys must be nonfunctional before reduction in renal function is severe enough to be associated with significant elevations in either substance.

d. It is obvious that renal disease can occur without renal failure and uremia. Unfortunately, many renal diseases escape detection until they become so generalized that they induce clinical signs as the result of serious impairment of renal function.

D. RENAL FAILURE (Renal Insufficiency)

1. Renal failure implies that two-thirds to three-fourths or more of the functional capacity of the nephrons of both kidneys has been impaired. It may or may not be of sufficient severity to cause uremia.

a. In dogs, impaired ability to concentrate and dilute urine caused by renal disease cannot readily be detected until the functional capacity of about two-thirds of the nephrons of both kidneys is affected.

b. Renal azotemia and retention of other metabolites normally excreted by the kidneys are usually not recognized until the functional capacity of about 70 to 75% of the nephrons is affected.

2. The term renal failure is analogous to liver failure or heart failure in that a level of organ dysfunction is described rather than a specific disease entity.

3. Renal failure may be precipitated by acute or chronic, reversible or irreversible, prerenal, renal or postrenal diseases. It may be associated with polyuria or oliguria.

4. Clinical signs of polysystemic disorders caused by abnormalities of water, electrolyte, acid-base, endocrine

and nutrient balance are not invariably present in patients with primary renal failure (*i.e.*, not all patients with primary renal failure are uremic). This is related, at least in part, to the tremendous reserve capacity of the kidneys and the ability of unaffected nephrons to undergo compensatory hypertrophy and hyperplasia.

   a. Renal function adequate for homeostasis does not require that all nephrons be functional.

   b. Polysystemic signs of renal failure (*i.e.*, uremia), including vomiting, diarrhea, depression, anorexia, dehydration and weight loss, usually do not occur until approximately 75% or more of the total nephron population have been functionally impaired.

5. In some instances, uremic crises may suddenly be precipitated by prerenal (*i.e.*, pancreatitis, foreign body gastroenteritis, congestive heart failure) or less commonly postrenal (urethral obstruction, displacement of urinary bladder into perineal hernia) disorders which occur in patients with previously compensated primary renal failure.

E. UREMIA

1. When the structural and functional integrity of both kidneys has been compromised to such a degree that polysystemic signs of renal failure become manifest clinically, a relatively predictable symptom complex called uremia appears, regardless of the underlying cause.

2. Uremia is characterized by multiple metabolic and phys-

iologic alterations that result from renal insufficiency. Renal insufficiency may be caused by a large number of disease processes (infection, ischemia, endogenous or exogenous toxins, anomalies, obstruction to urine outflow, hypercalcemia, immune-mediated disorders and trauma) which have in common impairment of at least three-fourths of the nephrons of both kidneys. Depending on the biological behavior of the disease in question, primary renal failure may be reversible or irreversible.

3. Clinical signs of uremia are not directly caused by renal lesions, but rather develop as a result of multiple metabolic deficits and excesses that develop as a result of decreased renal function caused by generalized renal lesions.

4. Clinical signs characteristic of uremia are manifestations of an interaction between:

   a. Autointoxication caused by:
     (1) Reduction of renal function below that required to clear plasma of metabolic waste products and to produce hormones.
     (2) Impaired ability to conserve vital metabolites in glomerular filtrate.
     (3) Reduced degradation and synthesis of hormones.

   b. The body's compensatory attempts to maintain homeostasis.

5. Signs caused by underlying renal lesions may also contribute to the spectrum of clinical findings.

VI. TERMS AND CONCEPTS RELATED TO BACTERIURIA

A. BACTERIURIA is defined as the presence of bacteria in urine. It is not synonymous with urinary tract infection because:

1. Bacteria that normally inhabit the urethra and genitalia in the absence of urinary tract infection may appear in urine that is obtained by either spontaneous voiding or catheterization.

2. Urine may be contaminated with bacteria after it is voided.

B. SIGNIFICANT BACTERIURIA: The term significant bacteriuria is used to distinguish between bacterial contaminants and bacterial pathogens.

1. A high bacterial count in a properly collected and cultured urine sample is indicative of urinary tract infection.

2. Small numbers of bacteria indicate contamination.

C. ASYMPTOMATIC (Covert) BACTERIURIA:

Asymptomatic bacteriuria is defined as significant bacteriuria which is unassociated with detectable signs or routine laboratory evidence of urinary tract disease. The infection is confined to the urine.

1. Results of widespread screening programs revealed that asymptomatic bacteriuria is common in human beings, especially women. It is more commonly observed in patients with recurrent infections.

2. The frequency of asymptomatic bacteriuria in dogs and cats is unknown, although it does occur.

3. There is evidence that bacterial infection of human kidneys need not be accompanied by the classic features of acute pyelonephritis. Abnormal renal function may exist for months before signs typical of pyelonephritis appear. Presumably the same situation could occur in animals. Early detection of asymptomatic bacteriuria and asymptomatic pyelonephritis is clinically important because renal damage can be stopped with appropriate therapy.

VII. DEFINITION OF SOME LESS COMMONLY USED TERMS

A. MELITURIA: the presence of any type sugar in urine.

B. TITRATABLE ACID: The net amount of acid (proton) lost in urine or conserved by the body is estimated by measuring the number of milliequivalents of alkali or acid necessary to titrate urine from an acid or alkaline reaction to the normal pH of blood. Usually it is determined on 24-hour urine collections, and is expressed in units of milliequivalents of acid or alkali needed to neutralize the urine excreted *per* day to pH = 7.4.

Table 4

General Priorities for Clinical Evaluation

I. COLLECT INFORMATION
  A. Define data to be collected
  B. Follow written protocol on all patients

II. DEFINE PROBLEM(S)
  A. Refine to highest degree of refinement
  B. Do not overstate problems

III. FORMULATE DIAGNOSTIC PLANS
  A. Verification of problem(s) is first priority:
    1. especially important for historical problems such as hematuria, polyuria, dysuria, *etc.*
    2. also of significance for transient or intermittent problems
  B. Localization of problem(s) to body system(s) or organ(s) is second priority
  C. Consider probable cause(s) as third priority:
    1. pathophysiology first (Damn It)
    2. specific cause(s) next

IV. FORMULATE PROGNOSIS

V. FORMULATE THERAPEUTIC PLANS
  A. Specific
  B. Supportive
  C. Symptomatic
  D. Palliative

VI. FORMULATE FOLLOW-UP PLANS

From: Osborne, C. A., and Finco, D. R. (1978).
Diagnostic Procedures in Urology: Use and Misuse.
In: *Proc. 45th Annual AAHA Meeting.*

Chapter 2. Diagnostic Perspectives

Table 5

Defining Problems at an Appropriate Level of Refinement

UNREFINED	REFINED
1. Palpable bladder mass 2. Hematuria 3. Dysuria 4. Proteinuria 5. Pyuria 6. Significant bacteriuria	Disease of the urinary bladder associated with: 1. Palpable mass 2. Primary or secondary infection of the urinary tract (bacteriuria) 3. Dysuria 4. Inflammation of the urinary tract (pyuria, proteinuria, hematuria)

Table 6

Properly Defined Versus Overstated Problems

PROPER DEFINITION	OVERSTATED
Disease of the urinary tract associated with: 1. Primary or secondary bacterial infection (significant bacteriuria) 2. Inflammation of the urinary tract (proteinuria, pyuria, hematuria)	Nephritis caused by bacterial infection and associated with inflammation

Diagnostic Perspectives

I. GENERAL PRIORITIES FOR CLINICAL INVESTIGATIONS

In our opinion the first steps in the diagnostic process must be to define and verify problems (Table 4). These are essential beginning steps because one must be able to define problems before they can be solved. Errors made in identification and verification of clinical problems may not only lead to fruitless pursuit of nonexistent disorders, but they may result in a costly and time-consuming series of diagnostic and therapeutic plans before errors are identified.

Following accurate definition and verification of problems from data collected from the history, physical examination, and laboratory or radiographic procedures where appropriate, a complete problem list should be constructed. Problems should be stated at their highest level of refinement, and should be defined in such a way that their refinement can be defended with reasonable certainty on the basis of current knowledge about the patient. Listed from the lowest to the highest level of refinement, problems may be defined as:

1. A clinical sign (dysuria, hematuria, polyuria, etc.);
2. An abnormal laboratory finding (pyuria, bacteriuria, leukocytosis, etc.), radiographic finding (enlarged kidney, displaced urinary bladder, etc.), etc.;
3. A pathophysiological syndrome (primary renal failure, urinary tract infections, urolithiasis, etc.); and,
4. A diagnostic entity (pyelonephritis, struvite urolithiasis, etc.).

Disciplined thought is required to construct a meaningful problem list (Tables 5 and 6). When integrating problems to their highest degree of refinement, it is important to consider that clinical manifestations of disease are usually a combination of:

1. Signs induced by the disease (such as bacteriuria associated with infection of the urinary tract), and
2. The body's compensatory response to these problems (such as pyuria and perhaps proteinuria and hematuria

caused by host inflammation to eradicate bacteriuria and repair damaged tissues).

Localization of problems should follow their definition and verification (see Table 2). For example, if a patient is examined because of gross hematuria, but no other abnormalities are initially identified, the problem should be listed as gross hematuria. Additional information is required to determine its location(s) (kidneys, ureters, urinary bladder, urethra, genital tract) and cause(s) (anomalies, neoplasia, infection, uroliths, exogenous or endogenous toxins, coagulopathies, etc.). In contrast, if hematuria occurs independent of micturition and is associated with a palpable lesion of the urethra, the problem might be defined as a urethral lesion associated with gross hematuria.

Following localization of problems to a body system or organ, it is useful to think of basic pathophysiologic mechanisms when trying to determine probable (rather than possible) causes of each problem. The acronym DAMN IT may be useful for this purpose (Table 7). One of the most frequent errors made by inexperienced diagnosticians is the premature consideration of specific disease entities without:

Table 7

"Damn It" Acronym of Pathophysiology

D	Degenerative disorders
A	Anomalies Autoimmunity
M	Metabolic Disorders
N	Neoplasia Nutritional Disorders
I	Inflammation (infection or noninfectious) Immune Disorders Iatrogenic Disorders Idiopathic Disorders
T	Toxicity (endogenous or exogenous) Trauma (external or internal)

Modified from: Osborne, C. A. (1975). The Transition of Quality Patient Care from an Art to a Science: The Problem-Oriented Concept. JAAHA, 11: 250.

1. Verifying the existence of problems, especially those identified by owners,
2. Localizing problems to the appropriate body system or organ, and
3. Considering basic pathophysiologic disease mechanisms that might be involved.

If one habitually by-passes these important components of problem-solving, one will become overly dependent on establishing diagnoses on the basis of previous experience, rather than developing the capacity to diagnose disease processes never personally encountered.

Following establishment of the most probable causes of a problem, appropriate diagnostic tests and procedures should be performed to prove (rule in) or disprove (eliminate) them.

II. WHEN URINALYSES ARE INDICATED

A. A complete urinalysis should be performed on *every* patient suspected of having disease of the urinary system in order to collect data which will help to verify or eliminate diagnostic possibilities formulated on the basis of observations obtained from the history and physical examination. Examples of findings associated with some urinary diseases include:

1. PRIMARY RENAL FAILURE: varying degrees of impaired ability to concentrate and dilute urine in response to appropriate stimuli; low pH.
2. RENAL DISEASE: casts, proteinuria, hematuria, pyuria, sometimes glucosuria, *etc.*
3. URINARY TRACT INFECTION: significant bacteriuria typically associated with varying degrees of pyuria, hematuria, and proteinuria.
4. RENAL TUBULAR ACIDOSIS: impaired ability to acidify urine in response to appropriate stimuli.
5. FANCONI SYNDROME: Normoglycemia, glucosuria, amino-aciduria, proteinuria, and renal tubular acidosis.
6. CYSTINURIA: precipitation of cystine crystals, especially in acid urine.
7. NEOPLASIA: occasional presence of exfoliated neoplastic cells in urine sediment.

B. Evaluations of urinalyses are also particularly helpful in problem definition and problem verification in patients with nonurinary disorders. Like complete blood counts, the results of urinalyses provide information about the integrity of many body systems. For this reason, it is our practice to include urinalyses and hemograms as a part of the initial evaluation (so-called minimum data base) of all patients with an illness of unknown cause that is of such a nature as to require hospitalization (or frequent evaluation as an outpatient if hospitalization is not feasible). Detection of abnormal findings by urinalysis may dictate the need for further evaluation. Because the results often indicate the body system(s) or organ(s) affected, they often influence selection of additional diagnostic tests or procedures. Examples of findings in urinalyses which may be associated with extraurinary diseases include:

1. DIABETES MELLITUS: hyperglycemia, glucosuria, sometimes ketonuria.
2. PITUITARY DIABETES INSIPIDUS: hyposthenuria.
3. HEPATIC DISEASE: bilirubinuria; sometimes ammonium urate, tyrosine, and other crystals.
4. SEVERE HEMOLYTIC DISEASE: hemoglobinuria, hyperurobilinogenuria.
5. PRERENAL AZOTEMIA: formation of concentrated urine (also called baruria or hypersthenuria).
6. SYSTEMIC ACIDOSIS (acidemia): frequently the formation of acid urine.

III. NORMAL VERSUS ABNORMAL RESULTS

Results of urinalyses provide information that help to evaluate the integrity of the urinary and other body systems. The value of test results that indicate an abnormality is obvious. Results of tests that indicate normalcy are also of great value. Normal findings indicate that selected physiologic processes governing formation of urine (including selective permeability of glomeruli, tubular reabsorption of some metabolites, and tubular secretion of others) are functioning adequately. Knowledge that physiologic processes are functioning adequately provides objective information with which to exclude them as a cause of the clinical signs.

Whether a particular value is normal or abnormal is often influenced by the condition of the patient at the time the sample was collected, the method of collection, the type (if any) of preservation used, the laboratory method used, and whether or not diagnostic or therapeutic agents were given prior to sample collection. Therefore, appropriate consideration of these variables is extremely important in interpreting test results.

IV. SERIAL URINALYSES

Single determinations of most laboratory tests indicate the status or functional competence of the organ or body system at the time the tests are performed. Single evaluation of many laboratory tests, including urinalyses, is analogous to obtaining a patient's temperature once. In such situations, it cannot be determined whether or not an abnormality is remaining static, increasing or decreasing in severity, nor

can the rate at which change is occurring be determined. Re-evaluation of appropriate components of urinalyses often indicates the trend of the abnormality. Detection of remission or exacerbation of abnormal test results by serially performed tests often provides a reliable index of prognosis, and/or the efficacy of treatment.

Chapter 3. Laboratory Considerations

Laboratory Considerations

I. OVERVIEW

Urinalyses may provide a great wealth of diagnostic information. Because of the complex nature of normal and abnormal urine, however, and because of rapid and unpredictable changes in urine composition that may occur following collection, analysis of this golden liquid is not a "routine" task that should be relegated to improperly trained personnel with no perspective of the need of standardization and precision in technique, quality control, and the conceptual difference between observations and interpretations. Although diagnostic analysis of urine is comparatively rapid and inexpensive, incorrect technique and overinterpretation or underinterpretation of test results may seriously hinder diagnostic efforts. Erroneous diagnostic information is often a greater stumbling block than lack of diagnostic information because it has a tendency to eliminate the search for correct information. The frightening outcome may be misdiagnosis, erroneous prognoses, and administration of ineffective or contraindicated therapy.

Like all laboratory tests, results of urinalyses are helpful, but not infallible. Their value is directly proportional to the diagnostician's ability to interpret them. Since the results of urinalyses are significantly influenced by biologic and technical factors, results should be interpreted in combination with available findings from the history and physical examination, and data from radiographic, biopsy and other laboratory procedures when available.

II. PROCEDURES FOR ROUTINE SCREENING URINALYSIS

A. Warm sample to room temperature if refrigerated.

B. Thoroughly mix sample.

C. Transfer 5 ml to a conical tip centrifuge tube. The remainder of the urine sample should be saved until all procedures are completed so that any of the tests can be repeated, if necessary, or other special tests can be performed.

D. Evaluate color and turbidity in the transparent centrifuge tube.

E. Immerse test portions of reagent strips into urine sample and rapidly remove. Gently tap edge of strips on the edge of collection container to remove excess urine. Compare color of various reagent pads to the color scale provided by the manufacturer at proper time intervals.

1. Ignore the nitrite test (if present).
2. If the test pad indicates proteinuria, verify its presence by repeating the procedure on urine supernatant. If the reaction for protein is still positive, verify reagent strip results with the sulfosalicylic acid test for proteinuria.
3. If the test pad indicates glucosuria, semiquantitate test results with the copper reduction method for glucosuria.
4. Evaluate the test for ketonuria.
5. Use care when interpreting the test for urobilinogen.
6. Evaluate the test for bilirubinuria.
7. If the test pad is positive for blood, repeating the test on urine supernatant may aid in differentiating hematuria from hemoglobinuria and myoglobinuria.

F. Determine urine specific gravity.

1. If a urinometer is used, ideally the temperature of the urine should correspond to reference temperature of the urinometer.
2. If a refractometer is used, evaluate uncentrifuged urine if it is clear. If it is turbid, centrifuge (as described in G) and use supernatant.

G. Centrifuge 5 ml of urine in a conical tip centrifuge tube for 3-5 minutes at 500-3000 RPM.

1. Remove the supernatant by decanting or with a rubber-topped disposable pipette, and save for potential chemical analysis. Allow a standard volume (approximately ½ ml) of supernatant to remain in the test tube.
2. Thoroughly resuspend the urine sediment in the remaining supernatant by agitation of the tube or by "finger flipping" of the tube.
3. Transfer a drop of reconstituted sediment to a microscope slide with a rubber-topped disposable pipette and place a coverslip over it.

4. Subdue the intensity of the microscope light by lowering the condenser and closing the iris diaphragm (or use a phase microscope).

5. Systematically examine the entire specimen under the coverslip with the low power objective, assessing the quality and type (casts, cells, crystals, *etc.*) of sediment.

6. Examine the sediment with the high power objective to identify the morphology of elements and to detect bacteria.

H. Record the results.

III. QUALITY CONTROL

A. Positive and negative control samples of urine (Tek-Chek®, Urintrol®, Kovatrol®) may be purchased to evaluate some test procedures of routine urinalyses (*see* Appendix: Ames Co., Harleco and ICL Scientific, respectively).

1. Control material may be either urine (lyophilized pooled human urine) or an aqueous solution with various ingredients adjusted to desired concentrations:

   a. The products usually have long-term stability in lyophilized form.

   b. The products usually have limited stability following reconstitution.

   c. Assayed values are provided with each product.

2. Control reagents can be utilized as blind samples (unknown) or as control specimens (known).

B. Questions about the reliability of a specific manufacturer's lot of reagent strips or tablets may sometimes be answered by repeating the test(s) with new reagents from a different lot number.

C. Urinometers and refractometers should be periodically checked for accuracy with solutions of known specific gravity.

D. Development of expertise in recognition of red cells and white cells in urine sediment may be facilitated by adding blood to normal urine and examining the sediment. Similarly, transitional epithelium may be harvested from blood donors with the aid of a catheter, or at necropsy, and added to normal urine prior to preparation of sediment.

IV. DRUG-INDUCED ERRORS OF ROUTINE URINALYSES

A. OVERVIEW

1. Because drugs may alter laboratory test values by a variety of pharmacologic, physical, and/or chemical mechanisms, urine samples should be collected prior to administration of diagnostic and therapeutic agents.

2. If therapy has been given prior to sample collection, the time and sequence of therapy and sampling should be recorded in order to facilitate meaningful interpretation of results.

B. FLUIDS AND DIURETICS

1. Oral or parenteral administration of fluids or diuretics may alter urine specific gravity and osmolality.

2. Therapeutic dosages of furosemide may cause urine to become acid.

3. Increased urine volume may suppress positive test results by dilution of reactants.

4. Dilute urine (urine specific gravity < 1.008) often causes varying degrees of cell lysis.

5. Administration of parenteral solutions containing glucose may cause varying degrees of glucosuria and diuresis.

C. ANTIMICROBIAL AGENTS

1. Urine for culture should be collected prior to administration of antimicrobial agents. In instances where diagnostic culture is needed following initiation of antimicrobial therapy, we suggest that therapy be withdrawn for three to five days before samples for culture are collected.

2. High doses of carbenicillin and benzyl-penicillin have been reported to cause an increase in urine specific gravity in human beings.

3. Release of formaldehyde from methanamine may inhibit glucose oxidase and peroxidase systems utilized in some glucose and occult blood, hemoglobin, and myoglobin determinations. Formaldehyde may also interfere with tests for urobilinogen.

4. Large doses of penicillin, cephaloridine, and sulfisoxazole have been reported to give a false positive reaction for protein detected by sulfosalicylic acid.

D. ACIDIFIERS AND ALKALINIZERS

1. Administration of acidifiers or alkalinizers may alter crystal composition in addition to urine pH.

2. Highly alkaline urine samples may induce false positive reactions for protein detected by commonly used reagent strips and false negative reactions with sulfosalicylic acid.

3. Ascorbic acid may cause a false positive reaction for glucose detected by copper reduction methods, and a false

negative reaction for glucose detected by glucose oxidase methods.

4. Ascorbic acid may also inhibit reduction of nitrate to nitrate and chemical tests for red cells, hemoglobin and myoglobin.

E. RADIOPAQUE CONTRAST AGENTS

1. Commonly used triiodinated radiopaque contrast agents may alter urine specific gravity and osmolality.

    a. If the preadministration urine sample has a specific gravity *below* approximately 1.040, the specific gravity will typically rise following urinary excretion of radiopaque contrast agents.

    b. If the preadministration urine sample has a specific gravity *above* approximately 1.040, the specific gravity will typically fall following urinary excretion of radiopaque contrast agents (possibly as a result of osmotic diuresis).

2. Triiodinated radiopaque contrast agents may induce false positive reactions for protein detected by sulfosalicylic acid (refer to Chapter 7, CHEMICAL CHARACTERISTICS, Table 14).

F. Consult the discussion of specific tests of routine urinalyses for additional information about drug-induced errors of results.

V. TIMING OF ANALYSIS

A. Urine obtained at any time may be satisfactory for screening analysis; however, the composition of urine may vary considerably throughout the day.

B. There are advantages to collection of urine for analysis during specific periods.

1. EARLY MORNING (OR FASTING) SAMPLES:

    a. Advantages
        (1) Most likely to be concentrated, and therefore facilitates evaluation of tubular capacity to concentrate urine without special techniques.
        (2) Most likely to contain higher yield of cells, casts, and bacteria because:
            (a) of duration of formation.
            (b) likely to be acid (an acid pH tends to prevent dissolution of proteinaceous structures).
            (c) of concentration (dilute urine promotes lysis of cells).

    b. Disadvantages
        (1) Less likely to reveal hyperglycemic glucosuria than a 1-3 hr postprandial sample.
        (2) Cytology of cells likely to be altered by prolonged exposure to wide variations in pH and osmolality and waste products.

2. RECENTLY FORMED SAMPLES:

    a. Advantages
        (1) Cytologic detail often superior to samples stored in bladder for several hours.
        (2) Fastidious bacteria inhibited by urine may be easier to detect.

    b. Disadvantages
        (1) Sample may not be sufficiently concentrated to permit evaluation of tubular function.
        (2) Dilute samples may cause lysis or distortion of cells (especially RBC and white cells).

VI. SAMPLE PRESERVATION

A. INSTABILITY OF URINE

Urine is an unpredictably unstable mixture, especially at high temperatures and in an alkaline environment. For this reason, it is recommended that urine samples be examined as soon as possible following collection (especially if it is alkaline) to eliminate unknown and unpredictable variables.

The objective is to analyze samples whose *in vitro* characteristics are similar to their *in vivo* characteristics.

1. In general, the longer the delay between the time of urine collection and the time of analysis, the less reliable are the results.

2. Exactly how long samples can be maintained at room temperature without significantly affecting their composition is unknown.

    a. One of the most detrimental alterations that occurs when urine is allowed to remain at room temperature following collection is a variable increase in pH, secondary to proliferation of urease-producing bacterial contaminants, and escape of CO_2 from urine into the atmosphere. Alkaline urine promotes lysis of red cells, casts, and especially white cells, and may alter crystal composition as well.

    b. Cells may undergo osmotically-induced lysis in dilute (SG less than approximately 1.008) urine samples.

3. Most agree that samples should be analyzed within 30 minutes from the time of collection. Otherwise some form of preservation (usually refrigeration) should be considered.

4. In order to aid in meaningful interpretation of results, the time of collection and the time of analysis should be recorded independently on the urinalysis form (*see* Figure 1).

B. FRESHLY-FORMED VS. FRESHLY-VOIDED OR COLLECTED URINE

1. Freshly-formed urine is not necessarily synonymous with freshly-voided urine or collected urine.

2. Urine stored in the urinary bladder for several hours may change in composition.

   a. From a diagnostic standpoint, this generality is especially applicable to casts, cells, bacteria, and perhaps pH and crystals.

   b. Growth of bacteria may be enhanced or inhibited, depending on the species of bacteria and composition of urine.

   c. Bacteria themselves may alter the concentration of metabolites such as glucose.

3. Consult preceding section, Timing of Analysis, for additional considerations.

C. GENERALITIES CONCERNING URINE PRE-SERVATIVES

1. The objective of all preservation procedures is to prevent or minimize alterations in physical and chemical properties of urine, and to minimize changes in cells, casts, crystals, and organisms.

2. Urine specimens should be protected from exposure to intense light, especially sunlight, because some metabolites (such as bilirubin) may be rendered undetectable.

3. There is no universal preservative satisfactory for all tests of routine urinalyses.

   a. Bacteriostatic and bacteriocidal agents may interfere with one or more chemical and enzyme tests.

   b. Acidifying agents may alter crystals.

   c. Freezing may destroy cells and casts.

   d. Addition of a significant volume of preservative in proportion to the volume of the urine sample will interfere with semi-quantitation of results as a result of dilution.

   e. Ascorbic acid in concentrations of approximately 100 mg/dl prevents oxidation of bilirubin, but ascorbic acid in concentrations greater than 20 mg/dl interferes with methods utilizing glucose oxidase to detect glucose.

4. Some perspective on the alterations that occur during refrigeration may be obtained by comparing results of the pH and chemical composition of the sample as determined with diagnostic strips (Chemstrip® and Multistix®) before and after refrigeration.

5. If preservatives for urine sediment are used, consider dividing the sample into two aliquots of appropriate size.

   a. Add an appropriate quantity of preservative to that portion saved for sediment examination.

   b. Do not add preservative to the aliquot saved for chemical analysis.

6. Consult the following information for effects that commonly-used preservatives have on various tests.

7. If it is suspected that a preservative might be needed for a special procedure, consult the laboratory that is to perform the test for specific instructions on which preservative to use (if any).

D. REFRIGERATION

1. If it is known that analysis of a urine specimen will not be performed within 30 minutes from the time of its collection, the sample should be immediately refrigerated (2-8°C). The yield of RBC, WBC, and casts in unrefrigerated samples (especially if alkaline and/or dilute) will be inaccurate within a few hours following collection.

2. The length of time that various components of canine and feline urine samples will remain unaltered, or will undergo minimal alteration, during refrigeration has not been determined under controlled conditions. Uncontrolled clinical impressions have been interpreted by most investigators to indicate that the sample may be preserved for several hours, and possibly overnight. Consider the results of studies performed on refrigerated human urine:

   a. Red blood cells remained stable in refrigerated *acid* urine for several days.

   b. White blood cells remained stable in refrigerated *alkaline* urine for approximately three days, and in refrigerated *acid* urine for more than ten days.

3. Until more refined data become available, we cautiously

suggest that refrigerated urine is suitable for examination after several hours. If no alternative exists, it may be used for examination after twelve hours.

4. Samples should be stored in containers with tight-fitting lids to minimize evaporation.

5. Urine samples should be warmed to room temperature prior to analysis.

    a. Enzyme-based tests (glucose oxidase) require that urine samples be at room temperature (especially those designed to be evaluated ten seconds after contacting urine).

    b. The specific gravity of cold urine is higher than warm urine (consult Chapter 6, discussion on urinometers).

    c. Precipitated substances are more likely to redissolve in samples that have been rewarmed.

E. FREEZING

1. Freezing is a satisfactory method of preserving urine for most chemical reactions since it inhibits bacterial growth and retards decomposition of most metabolites.

2. Freezing is not a satisfactory method for preserving samples for sediment examination since it will cause varying degrees of cellular disruption.

3. Freezing is a satisfactory method of preserving the following metabolites for at least ten weeks: calcium, sodium, potassium, chloride, magnesium, and phosphate.

4. Significant losses of the following metabolites may occur following freezing: antidiuretic hormone, creatinine, epinephrine, hydroxyproline, norepinephrine, and urea nitrogen.

5. Frozen samples should be stored in tightly-closed containers to minimize evaporation.

6. Depending on the laboratory test to be performed, it may be important to rewarm the sample to promote solution of precipitated substances, and/or to facilitate the reaction of enzyme-based tests.

F. ACIDIFICATION

1. Cells, casts and some chemical constituents may be preserved for a short time by acidifying urine, especially if it is alkaline.

2. Crystals normally found in alkaline urine will tend to dissolve after acidification, while crystals found in acid urine will tend to form.

3. Procedure for sediment:

    a. Determine urine pH.

    b. If neutral or alkaline, add 0.1 normal HCl dropwise until the pH becomes acid.

4. Procedure for chemical constituents:

    a. A sufficient quantity of HCl is added to bring the specimen to a pH of 1 to 2 (usually 1 ml of 0.1 normal HCl per 100 ml urine).

    b. For 24-hour collections, the collection container should contain approximately 10 ml HCl.

    c. Urine preserved with HCl may be used for analysis of δ-amino-levulinic acid, catecholamines, estradiol, estrogens, estrone, and hydroxyproline.

5. Preservation of urine for amino acid analysis may be accomplished by adding drops of one normal hydrochloride until a pH of 3 is reached. The sample should then be frozen.

G. FORMALDEHYDE

1. Formaldehyde prevents microbial growth and aids in preservation of casts and cells.

2. One drop of 40% formalin *per* 30 ml of urine is adequate. Mixing of 20 ml of urine with 40 ml of 4% formaldehyde in water has also been reported to provide good results.

3. Formaldehyde interferes with the determination of glucose by techniques utilizing glucose oxidase.

H. THYMOL

1. Thymol is usually used as an antimicrobial preservative.

2. Thymol will induce false positive reactions for protein if sulfosalicylic acid or Exton's reagent is used.

3. Thymol is added to urine as a 10% (W/V) solution in isopropanol. Five to ten mls is sufficient to preserve a 24-hour urine collection from an average-sized dog.

I. TOLUENE

1. Toluene prevents microbial growth when added in sufficient quantities to saturate urine.

2. Toluene will help to prevent loss of acetone, but will alter the quantity of acetone detected since acetone is half as soluble in toluene as in water.

3. Toluene is a solvent, and may dissolve cups and other collection containers composed of synthetic material.

4. A quantity sufficient to form a film over the top of the urine in the collection container is adequate.

5. The portion of the urine specimen to be examined should be collected from beneath the surface layer of toluene.

J. CHLOROFORM

1. Chloroform is an antimicrobial preservative when added in sufficient quantities to saturate urine.
2. Five ml of chloroform is adequate to preserve a 24-hour urine sample obtained from an average-sized dog.

K. BORIC ACID

Boric acid at a concentration of 0.8% (¼ saturation) has been reported to be superior to formaldehyde, chloroform, and toluene in inhibiting bacterial growth. However, some bacterial growth may occur.

1. One gram of boric acid is adequate to preserve a 24-hour sample.
2. Urine preserved with boric acid may be used for analysis of androsterone, chorionic gonadotropin, dehydro-epiandrosterone, 17-ketogenic steroids, pituitary gonado-tropins, pregnanediol, pregnanetriol, 5-hydroxyindole acetic acid, and vanillylmandelic acid.

L. METAPHOSPHORIC ACID (HPO_3)

1. Metaphosphoric acid may be used to preserve vitamin C.
2. An aqueous solution of 10% metaphosphoric acid is used. One volume of acid is added to five volumes of urine.

VII. DO'S AND DON'TS IN TECHNIQUE AND INTERPRETATION

A. DO store commercial reagents in a cool, dry place (not a refrigerator).
B. DO keep reagents away from moisture, direct sunlight, heat, acids, alkalis, and volatile fumes.
C. DON'T administer diagnostic or therapeutic agents prior to collection of urine for screening diagnostic tests.
D. DO make every effort to collect and analyze a urine specimen whose *in vitro* characteristics are similar to its *in vivo* characteristics.
E. DO minimize variations in results for your laboratory by consistently performing all steps in analysis of urine in a standard fashion.
F. DO use a urine quality control system.
G. DO rewarm refrigerated urine to room temperature before analysis.
H. DO evaluate test results at times specified by the manufacturer.
I. DON'T prepare urine sediment by centrifugation at excessive speeds.
J. DO record test results in an orderly fashion immediately after they are obtained (*see* Figure 1).
K. DO consider the method of urine collection and urine specific gravity before interpreting the significance of test results.
L. DO use caution in interpretation of results. Remember, the reliability and specificity of many commercially-manufactured tests for human beings have not been evaluated in animals under controlled conditions.

Chapter 4. Collection of Urine

Collection of Urine

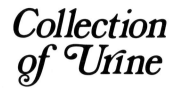

I. INTRODUCTION

The goal of urine collection is to procure a urine sample whose *in vitro* characteristics are similar to its *in vivo* characteristics. In addition to various tests, the method of collection and the collection container itself influence results and interpretation. In fact, knowledge of the method of collection is an essential prerequisite to interpretation of findings, such as hematuria, pyuria and bacteriuria.

While in pursuit of a diagnosis, one must not create additional problems. Patients must be protected from iatrogenic complications associated with collection techniques, including trauma to the urinary tract and urinary tract infections.

II. COLLECTION CONTAINERS

A. Disposable and reusable containers designed specifically for collection of urine from human beings may be obtained from a variety of medical supply houses.

B. We routinely use disposable plastic cups designed for ice cream, *etc.*
   1. These cups are clean, readily available, inexpensive and have tight-fitting lids. They also permit complete immersion of diagnostic dipsticks.
   2. They may be sterilized with ethylene oxide gas.

C. Use of containers improvised by owners should be discouraged since they often contain contaminants (detergents, food, cosmetics, *etc.*) that may interfere with enzymatic and chemical tests.

D. Use of transparent containers made of glass or plastic facilitates observation of macroscopic characteristics of urine. If urinalysis cannot be performed within 30 minutes following collection, however, opaque containers or containers made of amber glass should be considered to minimize photochemical degradation of urine constituents by bright light.

E. Urine obtained for bacterial culture must be collected in sterilized containers with tight-fitting lids. Sterilized containers may be obtained by:
   1. Sterilizing Dixie® cups in ethylene oxide gas.
   2. Sterilizing glass or metal drinking cups in an autoclave.
   3. Purchasing them from commercial manufacturers.

F. Samples collected by catheterization or cystocentesis may be transported and stored in the collection syringe.

III. COLLECTION TECHNIQUES

A. Urine may be removed from the bladder by one of four methods:
   1. Natural micturition.
   2. Manual compression of the urinary bladder.
   3. Catheterization.
   4. Cystocentesis.

B. Regardless of the method used, meticulous technique should be used to:
   1. Prevent iatrogenic trauma to the urethra and urinary bladder.
   2. Prevent iatrogenic urinary tract infection.

IV. NORMAL MICTURITION

A. The primary advantages of this technique are that:
   1. It is not associated with any risk of complications to the patient.
   2. It can be used by clients.

B. The primary disadvantages of this method are:
   1. Samples may be contaminated with cells, bacteria, and other debris located in the genital tract or on the skin and hair.
   2. The patient will not always micturate at the will of the veterinarian.

C. This method is very satisfactory for routine urinalyses performed to screen patients for abnormalities of the urinary tract and other body systems. Depending on specific circumstances, however, it may be necessary to repeat analysis of a urine sample obtained by catheterization or cystocentesis. As a generality, samples collected from dogs by this method are less desirable for bacterial culture than samples collected by catheterization or cystocentesis.

D. When possible, the first portion of the urine stream should be excluded from the sample submitted for analysis because it may be contaminated during contact with the genital tract, skin and hair. In order to facilitate this recommendation, two cups may be used to collect the sample.

1. The portion of the sample collected in the second cup, when available, represents a midstream sample; the sample in the first cup may be discarded or used as an aid to detect suspected urethritis or genital tract disorders.

2. If technical difficulties or lack of patient cooperation prevent collection of the sample in the second cup, the sample in the first cup is still available for urinalysis. Such a sample obtained from dogs, however, may provide misleading results if used for quantitative bacterial culture.

V. MANUAL COMPRESSION OF THE URINARY BLADDER

A. Induction of micturition by application of digital pressure to the urinary bladder through the abdominal wall may be used to collect urine samples from dogs and cats.

B. The primary advantages of this procedure are:
1. The risk of iatrogenic urinary tract infection and iatrogenic trauma is minimal.
2. Urine samples may be collected from patients with distended urinary bladders at the convenience of the clinician.

C. The primary disadvantages of this procedure are:
1. The urinary bladder may be traumatized if excessive digital pressure is used. This is not only detrimental to the patient; the associated hematuria may interfere with interpretation of results.
2. The urinary bladder may not contain a sufficient volume of urine to facilitate this technique.
3. Samples are frequently contaminated with cells, bacteria, and other debris located in the genital tract, or on the skin and hair.
4. Micturition may be difficult to induce in some patients, especially male cats.
5. Bladder urine contaminated or infected with bacteria may be forced into the ureters, renal pelves and kidneys. Unlike normal micturition where detrusor contraction is associated with a coordinated relaxation of voluntary and involuntary urethral sphincters, manual compression of the bladder increases intravesical pressure, but may not be associated with simultaneous relaxation of the urethral sphincters.

D. Technique.
1. Obtain appropriate information to be sure that complete obstruction of the urethra does not exist.

2. Outline the urinary bladder by abdominal palpation. As a generality, this technique will not be successful in the conscious patient unless the bladder contains at least 15 ml of urine.

3. The patient may be in a standing or recumbent position.

4. Exert moderate digital pressure over as large an area of the bladder as possible with the fingers and thumb of one hand, or with the fingers of both hands.

   a. Try to direct the force towards the neck of the urinary bladder.

   b. Steady continuous pressure should be applied rather than forceful intermittent squeezing motions.

   c. Avoid vigorous palpation and/or excessive pressure since the latter often causes iatrogenic hematuria.

   d. Sustain moderate digital pressure until the urethral sphincters relax and urine is expelled from the bladder. Several minutes of digital pressure may be required before micturition is induced.

   e. Avoid use of excessive pressure.

5. If the bladder is overdistended with urine because of partial obstruction to urine outflow, caution must be used not to rupture the bladder or urethra.

6. Although diuretics such as furosemide have been recommended by some investigators to facilitate collection of urine samples by increasing urine formation, alteration of urine specific gravity and pH is a notable drawback of this procedure. Use of diuretics to enhance urine collection by augmenting urine flow is therefore best suited for serial urine sample collections when dilution of urine is less critical (qualitative urine culture, *etc.*).

VI. CATHETERIZATION

A. OVERVIEW

1. Avoid unnecessary catheterization.
2. Catheterization should be performed in an atraumatic and aseptic fashion by persons familiar with the correct procedure. It is not a task which should be relegated to inadequately trained personnel who are unaware of the consequences of iatrogenic trauma and infection.

B. INDICATIONS

1. Diagnostic catheterization may be indicated to:
   a. Collect bladder urine for urinalysis or bacterial culture. There are times when catheterization is the only reliable means of obtaining a sample for diagnostic study.
   b. Collect accurately-timed volumes of urine for renal function studies.
   c. Monitor urine output in severely ill patients, in patients with urinary obstruction, or following urologic surgery.
   d. Instill contrast media for contrast radiography.
   e. Evaluate the urethral lumen for calculi, space-occupying lesions or strictures.
   f. Determine the volume of residual urine in patients with suspected neurogenic incontinence.
2. Therapeutic catheterization may be indicated to:
   a. Relieve obstruction to urine outflow.
   b. Instill medications into the urinary bladder.
   c. Facilitate surgical repair of the urethra or surrounding structures.

C. SIZE, COMPOSITION AND TYPES OF CATHETERS

1. SIZE

a. The scale of measurement commonly used for calibrating the diameter of catheters is the French scale (commonly abbreviated as F).
   (1) Each French unit is equivalent to $1/3$ mm; thus French units may be converted to millimeters by dividing by three.
   (2) A 9F catheter has an external diameter of 3 mm.
b. Catheters are available in a variety of diameters and lengths.

2. COMPOSITION

a. Urinary catheters are fabricated from a variety of materials including rubber, plastic, metal, nylon, latex and woven silk.
b. Catheters impregnated with radiopaque material are of value when used in conjunction with radiographic evaluation of the urinary system.
c. Catheters impregnated with antimicrobial agents have been recommended to minimize iatrogenic infection in human beings.

3. TYPES (Figures 2 and 3)

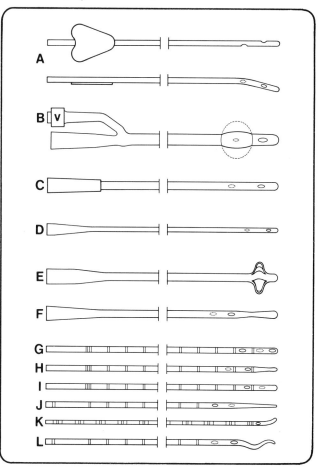

Fig. 2. Different types of catheters available for urine collection. A = rigid metal canine female urethral catheter; B = Foley self-retaining catheter with valve (v) for injection of air to inflate balloon (dotted circle); C = human urethral catheter with round tip; D = canine flexible urethral catheter; E = Malecot self-retaining four-winged catheter; F = olive tip human urethral catheter; G = whistle tip human ureteral catheter; H = olive tip human ureteral catheter; I = round tip human ureteral catheter; J = Blasucci flexible tip human ureteral catheter; K = Coude' tip human ureteral catheter; and L = Blasucci human ureteral catheter with flexible spiral filiform tip. Reprinted with permission of W. B. Saunders Company, Philadelphia, PA. From: *Canine and Feline Urology (2nd Ed., in preparation)*. By Osborne, C. A., Low, D. G., and Finco, D. R.

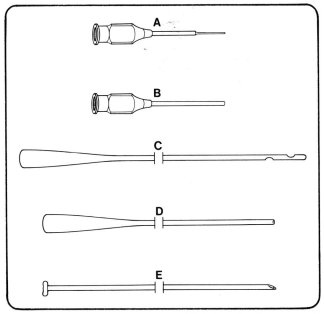

Fig. 3. Catheters used to collect urine and/or backflush the urethra of cats. A = rigid metal lacrimal cannula; B = silver abscess cannula; C = tomcat catheter; D = open end tomcat catheter; and E = intradermic polyethylene tubing with one end flared.

a. A wide variety of catheters (*see* Appendix: American Cystoscope Makers; C. R. Bard Inc.; Cutter Laboratories Inc.; Life-Tech Instruments Inc.) are available for use in human and veterinary medicine; each is designated to serve a particular need.

b. The openings adjacent to the tips of catheters are commonly called "eyes."
   (1) Catheters may have as few as one or as many as six or more eyes.
   (2) The edges of polypropylene catheters are sometimes rough and as a consequence irritate the mucosa of the bladder and urethra.

c. On the basis of the site of their insertion, human catheters have been classified as urethral or ureteral catheters.
   (1) Human urethral catheters are usually too large (and sometimes too short) for routine use in veterinary medicine.
   (2) Human ureteral catheters (*see* Appendix: American Cystoscope Makers; C. R. Bard Inc.; Cutter Laboratories Inc.; Life-Tech Instruments Inc.) are commonly used to catheterize male and female dogs.
   (3) Urethral catheters with inflatable balloons are called Foley catheters (*see* Appendix: American Cystoscope Makers; C. R. Bard Inc.; Cutter Laboratories Inc.; Life-Tech Instruments Inc.)

(a) By inflating the balloon following insertion of the catheter into the bladder, the tip of the catheter cannot migrate out of the bladder lumen.
(b) Foley catheters are designed to be used as in-dwelling (or retention) catheters.
(c) Pediatric Foley catheters are sometimes used for retrograde contrast urethrography and retrograde vaginography in dogs.

d. Canine urinary catheters.
   (1) Flexible plastic (*see* Appendix: Haver Lockhart Labs; Sherwood Medical Ind. Inc.) and rubber (*see* Appendix: Sherwood Medical Ind. Inc.) catheters similar in diameter and length to human ureteral catheters may be used to catheterize male or female dogs. Because they are relatively inflexible, polypropylene catheters frequently traumatize the urethras of male dogs as they curve around the ischial arch.
   (2) Metal catheters designed for use in female dogs are not recommended because their rigid structure frequently is the cause of iatrogenic trauma to the mucosa of the urethra and urinary bladder.
   (3) Swan Ganz flow directed balloon catheters (*see* Appendix: Edwards Laboratories) designed for human angiography are very useful for collection of quantitative urine specimens.

e. Feline urinary catheters (Figure 3).
   (1) Disposable polypropylene tomcat catheters (3½ to 5F) are available from commercial manufacturers (*see* Appendix: Sherwood Medical Ind.; Portex).
   (2) Infant feeding tubes (*see* Appendix: Sherwood Medical Ind.) and polyethylene tubing (*see* Appendix: Clay Adams Inc.) may also be used to catheterize cats.
   (3) Silver abscess cannulas (*see* Appendix: Becton Dickenson Co.) are often used to remove plugs from the distal urethra of male cats. They are too short to reach the lumen of the bladder.
   (4) The use of long rigid metal tomcat catheters is not recommended since they often cause trauma to the urethral and bladder mucosa.

f. It is recommended that a special drawer in the hospital be designated as a catheter drawer (analogous to a tool box).
   (1) Sterilized catheters of all sizes, composition and

types should be stored in this drawer, so that they will be readily available when needed.

(2) Speculums and light sources may also be stored in the catheter drawer.

D. CARE OF URINARY CATHETERS

1. Only sterilized catheters that are in excellent condition should be used.

   a. Catheters weakened during use or abuse may break apart while in the patient.

   b. The portion of the catheter where the "eye" is located is the weakest part of flexible catheters.

   c. Catheters that have a rough external surface may traumatize the mucosa of the urethra and urinary bladder. Not only are they detrimental to the patient; iatrogenic hematuria may interfere with interpretation of the urinalysis.

2. Catheters should be individually packaged prior to use. Use of transparent packaging material that may be sterilized by autoclaves (see Appendix: V. Mueller Co.) or ethylene oxide (see Appendix: American Hospital Supply) aids in storage and selection since it permits visualization of the catheter.

3. Nonsterilized catheters should never be used because:

   a. They may cause iatrogenic infection of the urinary system.

   b. They may contaminate urine that is collected for bacterial culture.

4. Sterilization:

   a. Catheters must be thoroughly cleansed prior to sterilization. Cleansing solutions should be thoroughly rinsed from them since they may interfere with enzymatic and chemical tests.

   b. Repeated autoclaving of nonmetal catheters may reduce their longevity.

   c. Ethylene oxide sterilization is excellent.

   d. Chemical sterilizing solutions containing quaternary ammonia compounds may be used, but are less effective than sterilization by autoclaving or ethylene oxide gas. In addition, if residual antiseptic solutions are not thoroughly rinsed from catheters they may:

      (1) Irritate the mucosa of the urethra or urinary bladder.

      (2) Interfere with growth of bacteria.

      (3) Alter chemical and enzyme tests.

   e. Disposable catheters, which are prepackaged in sterilized wrappers, may be obtained from commercial manufacturers.

E. POTENTIAL COMPLICATIONS

1. Discussion of potential complications precedes discussion of technique in order to emphasize the fact that catheterization of the urinary bladder is not an innocuous procedure.

2. TRAUMA

   a. Trauma to the urinary tract during catheterization can usually be avoided by selection of smooth flexible catheters and a good technique.

   b. Hematuria, associated with catheterization, usually indicates poor equipment or poor technique. Even meticulous technique, however, may induce bleeding if disease processes have markedly increased the vascular supply of the bladder and/or urethra. Cystocentesis may be considered in the latter instance.

   c. Although catheter-induced hematuria is usually self-limiting, it may interfere with interpretation of the results of urinalysis.

   d. Trauma to the urinary tract mucosa also predisposes the patient to bacterial infection since it damages normal host-defense mechanisms.

3. INFECTION

   a. A resident population of bacteria (primarily Gram positive *Staphylococci* and *Streptococci* along with Gram negative organisms) and mycoplasma are normally present in progressively increasing numbers from the mid-zone of the urethra to the distal urethra. Resident bacteria and mycoplasma are also present in the vagina and prepuce.

   b. Urine in the kidneys, ureters, and urinary bladder of normal dogs and cats is usually sterile. In addition to systemic natural defense mechanisms, the following local defense mechanisms are thought to prevent urinary tract infection in normal animals:

      (1) Normal micturition.

      (2) Normal anatomy.

      (3) Mucosal defense barriers.

      (4) Antibacterial properties of urine.

      (5) Renal defense mechanisms.

c. Catheterization, no matter how carefully executed, is always associated with the hazard of urinary tract infection because bacteria normally residing in the distal urethra are carried into the bladder.

d. The risk of bacterial infection caused by catheterization is dependent on the integrity of systemic and local host-defense mechanisms.

   (1) Provided proper technique is utilized, risk of bacterial infection following catheterization of a normal urinary bladder is low.

   (2) Catheterization of a patient with pre-existing disease in the urethra and/or urinary bladder is much more likely to be associated with iatrogenic infection. Cystocentesis should be considered for high-risk patients.

   (3) Repeated catheterization and indwelling catheterization should be avoided when possible since there is an increased risk of iatrogenic infection associated with these procedures.

e. Preventable causes of bacterial infection of the bladder associated with catheterization include:

   (1) Inadequate cleansing of periurethral tissues (prepuce, vagina, *etc.*).

   (2) Use of nonsterile equipment.

   (3) Catheter-induced trauma to the mucosa of the urethra and bladder.

f. Because of the risk of inducing infection of the bladder as a result of catheterization, indiscriminate use of this technique is condemned. This generally, however, must be kept in perspective. When necessary for diagnostic or therapeutic purposes, carefully executed catheterization of the urinary bladder should be performed without hesitation.

g. Procedures which may be used to reduce the incidence of iatrogenic infection following catheterization include:

   (1) Avoiding indiscriminate use of the technique.

   (2) Allowing only properly trained personnel to perform the procedure.

   (3) Irrigation of the bladder with antibacterial solutions (neomycin, furacin, polymyxin, *etc.*).

      (a) Because the effect of this procedure is transient, its prophylactic efficacy is questionable.

      (b) Only solutions which are known to be sterile should be used.

      (c) The volume of solution used should be sufficient to allow contact with all portions of the bladder mucosa.

      (d) Caution in the use of solutions is recommended since accumulations of large quantities of antimicrobial, acid or anesthetic agents within an inflamed urinary bladder may result in absorption and systemic toxicity.

   (4) Use of catheters impregnated with antibacterial agents designed for man.

   (5) Use of cystocentesis in patients with a high risk of infection because of an underlying disease process.

F. TECHNIQUE—GENERALITIES FOR MALE AND FEMALE DOGS AND CATS

1. Regardless of the specific procedure employed, meticulous aseptic and gentle "feather-touch" technique should be used to prevent damage to delicate tissues of the genital tract, urethra and urinary bladder.

2. As stated previously, only well-trained individuals who comprehend the potential consequences of iatrogenic trauma and urinary tract infection should be given the responsibility to catheterize the urethra and urinary bladder.

3. Conscious patients should be restrained by an assistant in order to minimize contamination of the catheter and trauma to the urethra.

4. Animals should be gently restrained in a comfortable position in order to minimize the possibility of sudden unexpected movement which may result in contamination of the catheter or trauma to the urinary tract. Some form of sedation may be required for male cats, and is usually required for female cats. Appropriate caution should be used so as not to use an agent that alters the diagnostic, physical or chemical composition of the urine.

5. Use the smallest diameter catheter which will permit the objective of catheterization.

6. Catheters with flared ends are recommended, especially if the length of the catheter is similar to or shorter than the length of the urethra.

   a. If the end is not flared, the catheter may migrate into the urethra to a point where it cannot be removed.

   b. Many commercially-prepared catheters have flared ends which will accommodate the tip of a syringe.

7. If a stylet is used in the catheter, it should be lubricated before it is inserted into the lumen of the catheter. If it is not lubricated, difficulty may be encountered in removing the stylet after the catheter is placed in the patient (especially male dogs).

8. If necessary, structures adjacent to the external urethral orifice may be cleansed with germicidal soap, water, and sterilized sponges. The soap and water mixture should be thoroughly removed by rinsing to prevent contamination of the urine sample. Soapy water may:

   a. Impart a cloudy appearance to the sample.

   b. Inhibit bacterial growth.

   c. Cause lysis of cells.

   d. Interfere with chemical and enzyme tests.

9. The distance from the external urethral orifice to the bladder neck should be "guesstimated" and mentally transposed to the catheter. This step will reduce the likelihood of traumatizing the bladder mucosa due to overinsertion of the catheter, and will prevent an over-inserted catheter from re-entering the urethra.

10. The tip of the catheter and adjacent portions should be liberally lubricated with sterilized aqueous lubricant.

   a. Proper lubrication of the catheter will minimize discomfort to the patient and catheter-induced trauma to the urethra.

   b. In man, coating the catheter with a large quantity of water-soluble lubricant containing an antibacterial agent has been reported to decrease the number of bacteria pushed into the bladder lumen.

11. Although usually unnecessary, local anesthesia may be induced with a topical anesthetic, such as lidocaine hydrochloride [Anestacon®] (see Appendix: Conal Pharmaceuticals Inc.).

12. Asepsis must be maintained throughout the procedure.

   a. The portion of the catheter that enters the urethral and bladder lumen should not be allowed to contact the hair or the skin of the patient or clinician.

   b. The catheter may be manipulated:

      (1) By holding the distal end only.

      (2) Through the packaging material in which it is contained.

      (3) With the aid of a sterilized pediatric hemostat.

      (4) With sterilized surgical gloves.

13. Never force the catheter through the urethra.

   a. If difficulty is encountered in inserting the catheter through the urethra, withdraw the catheter for a short distance and insert it again with a rotating motion.

   b. Injection of a sterilized aqueous lubricant (whose viscosity has been decreased by addition of sterilized water or saline) through the lumen of the catheter may be of value.

   c. If these steps are unsuccessful, a smaller-diameter catheter should be used.

14. The tip of the catheter should be positioned so that its eyes are located just beyond the junction of the neck of the bladder with the urethra. In most instances this may be accomplished by inserting the catheter approximately one inch beyond the point at which urine flows through the catheter lumen.

   a. This position may be verified by injection of known quantities of air through the catheter into an otherwise empty bladder. Inability to recover almost all of the air via aspiration indicates improper positioning of the catheter.

   b. Proper positioning of catheters facilitates removal of all of the urine from the bladder, and minimizes the possibility of catheter-induced trauma.

15. Urine may be aspirated from the bladder with the aid of a syringe.

   a. Aspiration must be gentle in order to prevent trauma to the bladder (or urethral) mucosa as a result of sucking it into the eyes of the catheter.

   b. Attempts to enhance urine flow through the catheter into the syringe by application of digital pressure to the bladder are not recommended as routine procedure since they increase the likelihood of catheter-induced damage to the bladder mucosa.

   c. Although we do not routinely use them, 2-way or 3-way valves will minimize inadvertent injection of bacteria into the bladder.

16. Unless desired for specific study, the first several milliliters of urine obtained via the catheter should be discarded since it may be contaminated with bacteria, debris, and cells from the genital tract and urethra.

17. In patients with a high risk of developing iatrogenic infection as a result of catheterization:

a. Sterilized solutions of antimicrobial drugs may be injected into the bladder lumen as a prophylactic measure.

b. Follow-up urinalyses of bacterial cultures should be evaluated several days later in an attempt to detect iatrogenic infection at a subclinical stage.

G. CATHETERIZATION OF MALE DOGS
(Figure 4)

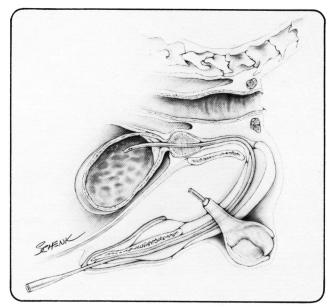

Fig. 4. Proper position of tip of flexible catheter in the lumen of the urinary bladder of a male dog. Rigid plastic catheters are often unsatisfactory because they cause trauma and pain during passage through the curved portion of the perineal urethra. Reprinted with permission of the American Animal Hospital Association. From: Techniques of Urine Collection; In: 44th Annual Proc. AAHA (1977). By Osborne, C. A., and Schenk, M. P.

1. Refer to general discussion about catheterization.
2. The diameter of the catheter will vary with the size of the patient. Four to 10 French catheters are satisfactory for most dogs.
3. The length of most human urethral and veterinary urethral catheters does not vary.
4. The external urethral orifice should be exposed by reflecting the prepuce away from the penis.

   a. Once exposed, the tip of the penis and the external urethral orifice should be rinsed with a cleansing solution.

   b. Once reflected, the prepuce must not be allowed to contact the catheter as it is being advanced through the urethral lumen.

5. Difficulty in advancing the catheter through the urethral

lumen may be encountered, especially at the level of the os penis and/or at the site where the urethra curves around the ischial arch.

6. Care must be used not to insert an excessive length of catheter because it may follow the curvature of the bladder wall, double back on itself, and re-enter the urethral lumen. A nonsurgical technique has been described to remove a catheter lodged in the urethra (Osborne *et al.,* 1972).

H. CATHETERIZATION OF FEMALE DOGS

1. Equipment (*see* Figures 2-3; Figure 5)

   a. Flexible veterinary urethral or human ureteral catheters identical to those used for male dogs are recommended. Rigid metal catheters are not recommended for routine use because they have a tendency to traumatize the mucosa of the vagina, urethra and urinary bladder.

   b. A variety of endoscopes may be used in the vagina to aid in visualization of the external urethral orifice, including (Figure 5):

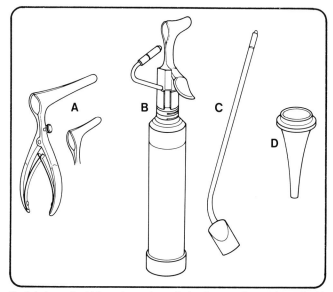

Fig. 5. Instruments which may be used as vaginal endoscopes. A = nasal specula with blades of different lengths; B = nasal specula with attached light source; C = transilluminator (without handle containing power source); D = otoscope head.

   (1) Human nasal specula.
   (2) Brincker-Hoff's human rectal speculum (small size).
   (3) Specula fashioned from disposable Monoject® syringe cases.
   (4) Pyrex® test tubes from which the end has been removed and the edge fire-polished.

(5) Otoscope cones.

(6) Laryngoscopes.

(7) Cystoscope sheaths.

   c. Transilluminator® (*see* Appendix: Welch-Allen) and light sources for otoscopes.

2. Refer to the general discussion about catheterization.

3. If necessary, remove excessive hair from around the vulva. Cleanse the perivulvar skin and vulva.

4. Flush the lumen of the vagina with sterilized water or saline injected through a syringe.

5. The external urethral orifice is located on a small tubercle in the ventral wall of the vagina.

   a. In the mature small- to medium-sized female dogs, the external urethral orifice is approximately 3-5 cm cranial to the ventral commissure of the vulva.

   b. The clitoral fossa lies just caudal to the external urethral orifice. Catheters and endoscopes inserted into the vagina must be carefully directed above and past this structure.

6. CATHETERIZATION *VIA* ENDOSCOPY (Figures 6-7)

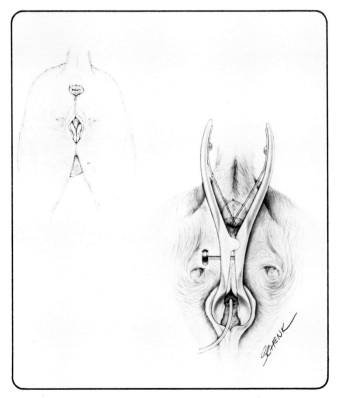

Fig. 6. Preferred position of nasal speculum used as vaginal endoscope to permit visualization of the external urethral orifice of female dogs.

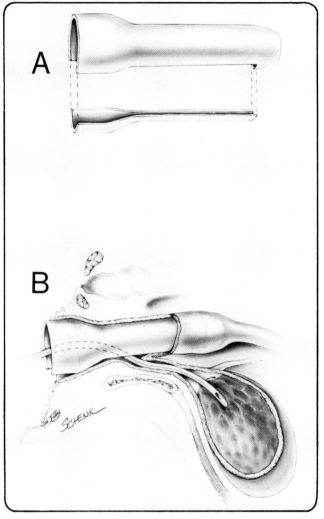

Fig. 7. Catherization of a female dog with the aid of an endoscope made from a Monoject disposable syringe container (Sherwood Medical Industries). The endoscope was made by removing a rectangular section from the side of the syringe case (A). Following insertion of the endoscope into the vagina with the open side positioned ventrally, a catheter can readily be directed into the external urethral orifice (B). Reprinted with permission of the American Animal Hospital Association. From: Techniques of Urine Collection; In: 44th Annual Proc. AAHA (1977). By Osborne, C. A., and Schenk, M. P.

   a. Good restraint, a good light source, and a comfortable position for both patient and clinician are important considerations.

   b. Having the dog in a standing position is recommended because it facilitates anatomical orientation required to locate the external urethral orifice.

   c. Ideally, the speculum should be large enough to remove most folds of the vaginal wall by distending its lumen.

   d. Injection of air into the vagina sometimes is of value in promoting dilation of its lumen.

7. FOLEY CATHETER TECHNIQUE

a. For patients too small to permit visualization of the external urethral orifice with the aid of an endoscope, an 8 to 10 F Foley catheter may facilitate catheterization.

b. Insert the Foley catheter into the vagina as far as possible and inflate the balloon.

c. Insert a small nasal speculum into the vagina and open the blades.

d. Gently pull the Foley catheter outward.

e. The urethral orifice may be visualized as a small opening in the ventral midline of the vaginal floor.

f. Insertion of the catheter through the urethral lumen will usually not be hindered by compression from the Foley balloon. If it is, however, the balloon should be deflated.

8. DIGITAL TECHNIQUE (Figure 8)

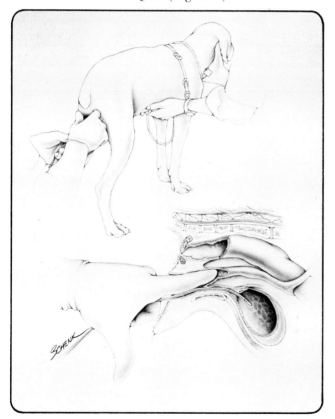

Fig. 8. Illustration depicting correct techniques of guiding flexible catheter into the external urethral orifice of a female dog. Keeping the patient in a standing position aids in anatomical orientation during blind digital palpation of the vaginal lumen. Reprinted with permission of W. B. Saunders Company, Philadelphia, PA. From: *Canine and Feline Urology (2nd Ed., in preparation)*. By Osborne, C. A., Low, D. G., and Finco, D. R.

a. Female dogs large enough to permit digital palpation of the vagina may be catheterized without need of direct visualization.

b. The dog should be standing as this facilitates anatomical orientation required to find the external urethral orifice. The external urethral orifice is located on the ventral midline of the vaginal floor.

c. Using sterilized gloves, the veterinarian should lubricate a finger and gently insert it into the vagina.

d. A sterilized flexible catheter should be inserted into the lumen of the vagina, dorsal to the clitoral fossa, and guided along the midline of the vaginal floor towards the external urethral orifice.

e. Although the external urethral orifice cannot be palpated, entry of the catheter into the urethra can readily be determined when the tip of the catheter disappears into the floor of the vagina.

f. The most common error of individuals inexperienced with this technique is overinsertion of the catheter into the vagina.

9. BLIND CATHETERIZATION (Figure 9)

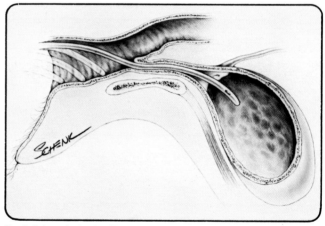

Fig. 9. Schematic drawing illustrating proper direction and curvature of a flexible catheter during blind advancement through the vaginal lumen into the external urethral orifice of a female dog. Reprinted with permission of W. B. Saunders Company, Philadelphia, PA. From: *Canine and Feline Urology (2nd Ed., in preparation)*. By Osborne, C. A., Low, D. G., and Finco, D. R.

a. This technique is usually more difficult than the methods previously described.

b. Blind catheterization may be useful in patients in which visualization or digital palpation of the external urethral orifice is not feasible because they are uncooperative or have a small vulvar orifice.

c. Because the position of the portion of the catheter within the vagina cannot be visualized, caution must be used to prevent trauma to the genital tract.

d. With the patient in a standing position to facilitate anatomical orientation, the lips of the vulva should be parted.

e. A sterilized, lubricated catheter should be inserted into the vagina and directed above the clitoral fossa.

f. With the long axis of the catheter directed in a cranioventral direction with respect to the long axis of the vagina, the tip of the catheter should be slowly advanced along the ventral midline of the vaginal floor.

g. The tip of the catheter must be kept on the ventral midline of the vaginal floor.

h. Detection of increased resistance to advancement of the catheter indicates that it has encountered the vaginal fornix. In this situation, the catheter should be withdrawn to a position just cranial to the clitoral fossa, and the procedure should be repeated.

i. Successful entry into the bladder may be detected by a lack of resistance to advancement of the catheter, and/or by passage of urine through its lumen.

I. CATHETERIZATION OF MALE CATS (Figure 10)

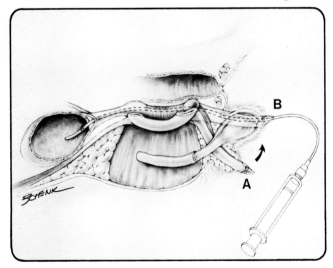

Fig. 10. Catheterization of a male cat. The penis has been extended from the preputial sheath by pulling it in a caudal position (A). The natural curvature of the caudal portion of the urethra is then minimized by displacing the extended penis in a dorsal direction, with the objective of aligning the long axis of the urethra with the long axis of the vertebral column (B). Reprinted with permission of the American Animal Hospital Association. From: Techniques of Urine Collection; In: 44th Annual Proc. AAHA (1977). By Osborne, C. A., and Schenk, M. P.

1. Equipment:

   a. Commercially-prepared flexible catheters that are 3 to 5 French in diameter are usually satisfactory.

   b. Catheters made from polyethylene tubing (*see* Appendix: Clay Adams Inc.) may be prepared by cutting one end at a 45° angle and flaring the other end with heat (Bunsen burner, match, *etc.*).

   c. Rigid metal catheters should be avoided as they often induce trauma to the urethral and vesical mucosa.

2. Refer to the general discussion about catheterization.

3. Although manual restraint by an assistant is usually satisfactory, sedation may be required for uncooperative cats. Appropriate caution should be used in selection of sedatives in order to prevent alteration of diagnostic, physical, and chemical components of urine.

4. Extend the penis from the preputial sheath by pulling it in a caudal direction.

5. Wash the end of the penis with a cleansing solution.

6. Displace the extended penis in a dorsal direction until the long axis of the urethra is approximately parallel to the vertebral column. This maneuver will facilitate atraumatic catheterization by reducing the natural curvature of the caudal portion of the urethra.

7. Gently insert the tip of the catheter into the external urethral orifice and advance it to the lumen of the urinary bladder.

8. Variable degrees of resistance may be encountered in normal cats because of the curvature of the urethra adjacent to the bony pelvis and/or voluntary contraction of skeletal muscle that surrounds the distal urethra. Resistance may be overcome by:

   a. Advancing the catheter with a rotating motion.

   b. Injecting a small quantity of sterilized isotonic fluid to distend the urethral lumen (*caution*—injection of fluids may alter test results).

9. Use care not to overinsert the catheter into the bladder lumen.

J. CATHETERIZATION OF FEMALE CATS

1. Equipment:

   a. Flexible catheters used for catheterization of male cats are satisfactory.

   b. Otoscope cones provide satisfactory vaginal endoscopes.

2. Refer to the general discussion about catheterization.

3. Some form of pharmacologic restraint is often required.

4. Carefully insert the tip of the catheter into the external urethral orifice located on the midline of the vaginal floor and advance it to the lumen of the urinary bladder.

VII. CYSTOCENTESIS (Figures 11 & 12)

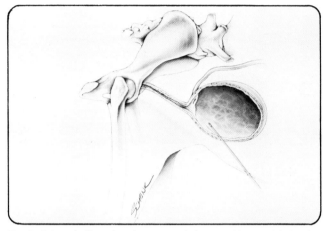

Fig. 11. Schematic illustration of cystocentesis in a cat. 22-gauge 3-inch spinal needle has been inserted through the ventral wall of the urinary bladder at an oblique angle. The point of insertion is several centimeters cranial to the junction of the bladder with the urethra. Reprinted with permission of the American Animal Hospital Association. From: Techniques of Urine Collection; In: 44th Annual Proc. AAHA (1977). By Osborne, C. A., and Schenk, M. P.

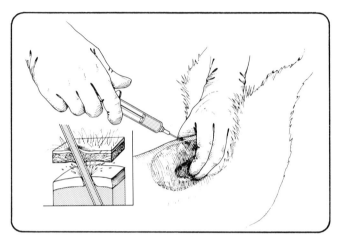

Fig. 12. Schematic drawing illustrating escape of urine through the bladder wall adjacent to the needle tract as a result of excessive digital pressure used to localize and immobilize the bladder. S = skin of abdominal wall; B = wall of urinary bladder. Reprinted with permission of W. B. Saunders Company, Philadelphia, PA...From: Cystocentesis. By Osborne, C. A., et al. In: Current Veterinary Therapy VII. (1980), Ed. R. W. Kirk.

A. Cystocentesis is a form of paracentesis consisting of needle puncture of the urinary bladder for the purpose of removing a variable quantity of urine by aspiration. Although techniques and complications of cystocentesis have not been evaluated by controlled studies, clinical experience has revealed that properly performed cystocentesis is of great diagnostic and therapeutic value. It is usually associated with less hazard of iatrogenic infection than catheterization and is often better tolerated by patients (especially cats and female dogs) than catheterization.

B. INDICATIONS

1. Diagnostic cystocentesis may be indicated to:

   a. Prevent contamination of urine samples with bacteria, cells and debris from the lower urogenital tract.

   b. Aid in localization of hematuria, pyuria and bacteriuria.

   c. Minimize iatrogenic urinary tract infection caused by catheterization, especially in patients with pre-existing diseases of the urethra and/or urinary bladder.

2. Therapeutic cystocentesis may be employed to provide temporary decompression of the excretory pathway of the urinary system when urethral obstruction or herniation of the urinary bladder prevents normal micturition.

C. CONTRAINDICATIONS

1. The main contraindications to cystocentesis are attempts to perform the procedure when there is an insufficient volume of urine in the urinary bladder, or when the patient resists restraint and abdominal palpation. Blind cystocentesis, performed without digital localization and immobilization of the urinary bladder, is usually unsuccessful, and may be associated with damage to the bladder or adjacent structures.

2. In our experience, collection of urine by cystocentesis from patients with bacterial urinary tract infection has not been associated with detectable spread of infection outside the urinary tract. In fact, collection of a urine sample for bacterial culture that has not been contaminated by passage through the urethra and genital tract is a frequent indication for cystocentesis.

D. EQUIPMENT

1. We routinely use 22-gauge needles. Depending on the

size of the patient and the distance of the ventral bladder wall from the ventral abdominal wall, 1½″ hypodermic or 3″ spinal needles (*see* Appendix: Becton Dickenson Co.) (Yale Spinal Needles) may be selected.

2. Small capacity (2½-12 ml) syringes are usually employed for diagnostic cystocentesis, while large capacity (20-60 ml) syringes are used for therapeutic cystocentesis. Alternatively, therapeutic cystocentesis may be performed with 6-12 ml syringes and a 2-way or 3-way valve (*see* Appendix: Pharmaseal Inc.).

E. SITE

1. Careful planning of the site and direction of needle puncture of the bladder wall is recommended. Although some clinicians recommend insertion of the needle into the dorsal wall of the bladder to minimize gravity dependent leakage of urine into the peritoneal cavity following withdrawal of the needle, we recommend that the needle be inserted in the ventral or ventrolateral wall of the bladder in order to minimize the chance of trauma to the ureters and major abdominal vessel (*see* Figure 11).

2. If therapeutic cystocentesis is to be performed, we recommend insertion of the needle a short distance cranial to the junction of the bladder with the urethra rather than at the vertex of the bladder. This will permit removal of urine and decompression of the bladder without need for re-insertion of the needle into the bladder lumen. If the needle is placed in, or adjacent to, the vertex of the bladder, it may not remain within the bladder lumen as the bladder progressively decreases in size following aspiration of urine.

3. We also recommend that the needle be directed through the bladder wall at approximately a 45° angle so that an oblique needle tract will be created (*see* Figure 11). By directing the needle through the bladder wall in an oblique fashion, the elasticity of the vesical musculature and the interlacing arrangement of individual muscle fibers will provide a better seal of the small pathway created by the needle when it is removed. In addition, subsequent distension of the bladder wall as the lumen refills with urine will tend to force the walls of the needle tract into apposition in a fashion somewhat analogous to the flap valve of the ureterovesical junction.

F. PRESAMPLING CONSIDERATIONS

1. Because insertion and withdrawal of a 22-gauge needle through the walls of the abdomen and bladder are associated with little discomfort, tranquilization, general anesthesia and local anesthesia are rarely required for diagnostic or therapeutic cystocentesis.

2. If the urinary bladder does not contain a sufficient volume of urine to permit digital localization and immobilization, the patient may be given oral fluids or a diuretic. Although diuretics such as furosemide may be used to facilitate the collection of urine samples by increasing urine formation, alteration of urine specific gravity and urine pH are notable drawbacks of this procedure. Even the quantity of bacteria *per* milliliter of urine may be significantly reduced, altering results of quantitative urine cultures. Use of diuretics to enhance urine collection by augmenting urine flow is therefore best suited for serial urine sample collections when information about urine specific gravity, urine pH and semiquantitative evaluation of routine test components is not significant.

G. TECHNIQUE

1. In order to perform cystocentesis without risk to the patient, deliberate planning of the site and direction of needle puncture is essential. The bladder must contain a sufficient volume of urine to permit immobilization and localization by palpation. Excessive hair should be removed with scissors or clippers. The ventral abdominal skin penetrated by the needle should be cleansed with an antiseptic solution each time cystocentesis is performed. Appropriate caution should be used to avoid iatrogenic trauma and/or infection of the urinary bladder and surrounding structures.

2. In cats, it is usually easiest to perform the procedure with the patient in lateral or dorsal recumbency. In dogs, the procedure may also be performed when the patient is standing.

3. Following localization and immobilization of the urinary bladder, the needle should be inserted through the ventral abdominal wall and advanced to the caudoventral aspect of the bladder. The needle should be inserted through the bladder wall at an oblique angle. If a large quantity of urine is to be aspirated, the needle should be directed so that it will enter the bladder lumen a short distance cranial to the junction of the bladder with the urethra. While the needle and bladder are immobilized, urine should be gently aspirated into the syringe. If a large quantity of urine is to be evacuated from the bladder, a 2-way or 3-way valve may be used.

4. Excessive digital pressure should not be applied to the bladder wall while the needle is in its lumen in order to prevent urine from being forced around the needle into the peritoneal cavity (*see* Figure 12). Use of a 3″ spinal needle rather than a 1½″ hypodermic needle when the ventral surface of the bladder wall is more than 1-1¼″ from the ventral abdominal wall permits immobilization of the urinary bladder without pulling it towards the ventral abdominal wall.

5. An appropriate quantity of urine for analysis and/or bacterial culture should be aspirated into the syringe. If disease of the bladder wall or virulence of urine pathogens is a likely cause of complications associated with loss of urine into the peritoneal cavity, the bladder should be emptied as completely as is consistent with atraumatic technique. These potential complications have not been a problem in our patients.

6. Use of prophylactic antibacterial therapy following cystocentesis must be determined on the basis of the status of the patient and retrospective evaluation of technique. In most instances, it is not required.

7. In order to minimize contamination of the peritoneal cavity with urine, unnecessary digital pressure should not be applied to the urinary bladder following cystocentesis.

H. PRECAUTIONS

1. We have not observed *ante mortem* post-biopsy complications in experimental or clinical studies in cats. Potential complications include damage to the bladder wall or adjacent structures with the needle, local or generalized peritonitis, vesicoperitoneal fistulas and adhesion of adjacent structures to the bladder wall.

2. We have encountered a few instances in which penetration of a loop of intestine by the needle resulted in false positive significant bacteriuria. Varying degrees of microscopic hematuria might be expected for a short period of time following cystocentesis, but are of little consequence since samples for laboratory analysis are rarely collected at this time.

Chapter 5. Physical Properties of Urine

Physical Properties of Urine

I. VOLUME

A. NORMAL

1. Normal urine volume is influenced by several variables including:
   a. Species.
   b. Body weight and size.
   c. Diet (especially water and salt content).
   d. Fluid intake.
   e. Physical activity.
   f. Environmental factors, such as temperature and humidity.

2. It has been estimated that normal adult dogs in a normal environment will produce approximately 12-20 ml of urine *per* pound of body weight *per* 24 hours.

3. In one study, normal adult cats produced on the average 8-9 ml of urine *per* pound of body weight *per* 24 hours.

4. Normal daily urine volumes for puppies and kittens have apparently not been determined.

B. INDICATIONS FOR DETERMINATION OF URINE VOLUME INCLUDE:

1. Verification of an observation of polyuria or oliguria.
2. Quantitation of substances excreted in urine (such as protein).
3. Evaluation of renal perfusion in patients with shock.

C. MEASUREMENT

1. Guesstimation of urine volume by observation of micturition is unreliable.
2. Use of metabolism cages provides more accurate data (*see* Chapter 1, section on Qualitative, Semiquantitative, and Quantitative Analyses, for further information).

3. Urine volume may be inferred from urine specific gravity:
   a. If the urine specific gravity of nonglucosuric urine samples is greater than 1.030, it is unlikely that polyuria exists. A specific gravity of this magnitude indicates that water is being reabsorbed from glomerular filtrate in excess of solute.
   b. If the urine specific gravity is below 1.030, any of the following might be present:
      (1) The patient could have physiologic polyuria.
      (2) The patient could have pathologic polyuria.
      (3) The patient could have pathologic oliguria.

D. POLYURIA (Table 8)

Table 8

Characteristic Urine Volumes Associated with Different Types of Azotemia in Dogs*

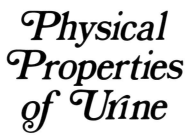

PRERENAL AZOTEMIA Physiologic oliguria (Dogs: $U_{SG} > 1.030$) (Cats: $U_{SG} > 1.035$) PRIMARY ACUTE ISCHEMIC OR NEPHROTOXIC AZOTEMIA Initial oliguric phase (Dogs: $U_{SG} = 1.007$ to 1.030) (Cats: $U_{SG} = 1.007$ to 1.035) Secondary polyuric phase (Dogs: $U_{SG} = 1.007$ to 1.030) (Cats: $U_{SG} = 1.007$ to 1.035)	OBSTRUCTIVE POSTRENAL AZOTEMIA Initial oliguria or anuria. Diuresis and polyuria following relief of obstruction. PRIMARY CHRONIC AZOTEMIA (Dogs: 1.007 to 1.030) (Cats: 1.007 to 1.035)* Terminal oliguric phase ($U_{SG} = 1.008$ to 1.012) Reversible oliguria may be caused by onset of nonrenal disorder that induces prerenal azotemia. (Dogs: $U_{SG} = 1.007$ to 1.030) (Cats: $U_{SG} = 1.007$ to 1.035)

*Urine specific gravity may become fixed between approximately 1.008 and 1.012 if sufficient nephron function is altered.
The specific gravity of glomerular filtrate is approximately 1.008 to 1.012.

1. Polyuria is defined as the formation and elimination of large quantities of urine.
   a. Depending on the body's need to conserve or eliminate water and/or solutes, polyuria may be normal (physiologic) or abnormal (pathologic).

b. The significance of polyuria without knowledge of additional information (history, physical examination, results of urinalyses, *etc.*) cannot be determined.

2. Physiologic polyuria.

    a. The most common cause of polyuria is physiologic polyuria.

    b. Physiologic polyuria usually occurs as a compensatory response to increased fluid intake.

    c. Proper evaluation of a patient with physiologic polyuria often requires a water deprivation or vasopressin response test.

3. Pharmacologic polyuria may occur:

    a. Following ingestion of sufficient quantities of salt to increase thirst.

    b. Following administration of diuretic agents.

    c. In dogs following administration of glucocorticoids (this appears to be a species-specific phenomenon).

    d. Following parenteral administration of fluids.

4. Pathologic polyuria.

    a. Polyuria may usually be classified as water diuresis or solute diuresis on the basis of examination of urine and blood.

    b. Water diuresis.

        (1) In general, water diuresis is characterized by a urine specific gravity and osmolality below (SG = 1.001 to 1.006; Osm = 50 to $\pm$ 150 mOsm/kg H_2O) that of glomerular filtrate (SG = 1.008 to 1.012; Osm = $\pm$ 300 mOsm/L).

        (2) Water diuresis results from lack of antidiuretic hormone (pituitary diabetes insipidus), decreased renal tubular response to adequate concentrations of antidiuretic hormone (renal diabetes insipidus), or excessive water consumption (psychogenic polydipsia).

    c. Solute diuresis.

        (1) In general, solute diuresis is characterized by a urine specific gravity and osmolality greater than that of glomerular filtrate.

        (2) Solute diuresis results from excretion of solute in excess of tubular capacity to absorb it (*i.e.*, glucose in diabetes mellitus), impaired tubular reabsorption of one or more solutes (*i.e.*, urea, creatinine, phosphorus and other solutes in pri-

mary renal failure), and/or abnormal reduction in medullary solute concentration that impairs the countercurrent system.

        (3) Disorders associated with pathologic polyuria and solute diuresis include chronic primary renal failure (*see* Table 8), the diuretic phase of acute renal failure (*see* Table 8), post-obstructive diuresis, hepatic disorders, and perhaps hyperadrenocorticism.

        (4) Polyuria, which occurs in association with clinical dehydration (caused by vomiting, diarrhea, *etc.*), indicates that the kidneys are unable to conserve water in spite of the body's need for water.

            (a) If renal function were normal, physiologic oliguria would be expected to occur as a compensatory response of the body to restore fluid balance.

            (b) Diseases that commonly, but not invariably, are associated with polyuria, vomiting and clinical dehydration include primary renal failure (regardless of cause), diabetic ketoacidosis, some cases of pyometra, and some cases with liver disorders.

            (c) Although polyuria, polydipsia and dehydration may be associated with diabetes insipidus, nephrogenic diabetes insipidus, hyperadrenocorticism, and primary polydipsia, these diseases are not typically associated with severe vomiting.

E. OLIGURIA

1. The term oliguria has been used to describe:

    a. States associated with decreased urine formation by kidneys.

    b. States associated with decreased elimination of urine from the body.

2. Oliguria associated with formation of a reduced quantity of urine is related to renal function and may be physiologic or pathologic in nature.

    a. Physiologic oliguria.

        (1) Physiologic oliguria occurs when normal kidneys conserve water in excess of solute in order to maintain or restore normal body fluid balance. Physiologic oliguria is characterized by the formation of a small volume of urine of high specific gravity.

(2) Urine production in patients with prerenal azotemia is a notable example of physiologic oliguria.

  (a) Prerenal azotemia is caused by abnormalities which reduce renal function by reducing renal perfusion with blood (*i.e.*, dehydration, shock, cardiac disease, hypoadrenocorticism). Since blood pressure provides the force necessary for glomerular filtration, marked decrease in blood pressure will result in reduction of glomerular filtrate. As a result, a variable degree of retention of substances normally filtered by glomeruli (urea, creatinine, phosphorus, *etc.*) results. In order to combat low perfusion pressure and reduced blood volume, the body secretes ADH to promote conservation of water filtered through glomeruli. Production of urine of high specific gravity, high osmolality, and low volume results.

  (b) Prerenal azotemia implies structurally normal kidneys which are initially capable of quantitatively normal function provided the prerenal cause is rapidly removed. If the prerenal cause is allowed to persist, primary ischemic renal disease may develop.

b. Pathologic oliguria.

(1) Pathologic oliguria usually occurs during the early phase of acute primary renal failure due to generalized ischemic or nephrotoxic tubular disease.

  (a) The exact pathophysiology involved in the production of oliguria in patients with acute nephrosis has not been established, although different mechanisms may be associated with different causes.

  (b) Available clinical and experimental evidence has been interpreted to suggest that marked reduction in glomerular filtration rate is an important factor. Obstruction of tubular lumens and abnormal reabsorption of filtrate through damaged tubular walls may also be involved in some cases.

  (c) The oliguria usually persists for hours to days, but in some instances its duration is so transient that it is not detected.

  (d) The specific gravity of urine (regardless of volume) obtained from patients with renal failure secondary to nephrosis will be similar to that of glomerular filtrate if a sufficient quantity of nephrons has been damaged to impair or prevent concentration and dilution of urine.

(2) An oliguric state may occur in a patient with primary polyuric renal failure if some prerenal abnormality (vomiting, decreased water consumption, cardiac decompensation, *etc.*) develops. If the prerenal cause is removed, and/or if proper fluid balance is restored, polyuria will resume.

(3) Oliguria may develop as a terminal event in patients with chronic progressive generalized renal disease.

3. Oliguria associated with elimination of a decreased volume of urine from the body is associated with diseases of the lower urinary system (ureters, urinary bladder, urethra) which impair flow of urine through the excretory pathway. Examples of diseases which impair urine outflow include:

a. Neoplasms, strictures or calculi which partially occlude the urethral lumen.

b. Herniation of the urinary bladder which partially obstructs urine outflow through the urethra, or urine inflow from the ureters.

F. ANURIA

1. The term anuria has been used to indicate the absence of urine formation by the kidneys, and absence of elimination of urine from the body.

2. Although it is possible that anuria could occur as a result of complete shutdown of renal function due to lack of renal perfusion of primary renal failure, it is usually associated with obstructive uropathy or rents in the lower urinary tract.

II. COLOR

A. OVERVIEW

Because of ease and lack of expense, determination of urine color is included in the routine complete urinalysis.

1. Caution must be used not to overinterpret the significance of urine color. Care should be taken to differentiate color from transparency.

a. Significant disease may exist when urine is normal in color.

b. Abnormal colors of the same type may be caused by several endogenous or exogenous pigments. Although they indicate an abnormality, they provide relatively nonspecific information.

2. Knowledge of urine color may also be of importance since it may induce varying degrees of interference with colorimetric test results.

3. Because the intensity of colors is dependent on the quantity of water in which associated pigments are excreted, it should be interpreted in light of urine specific gravity (no pun intended).

4. Detection of abnormal urine color should prompt questions related to diet, administration of medications, and environment.

5. Causes of abnormal colors should be substantiated with appropriate laboratory tests and examination of urine sediment.

B. NORMAL URINE COLOR

1. Normal urine is typically transparent light yellow, yellow or amber.

2. The yellow coloration is imparted primarily by two pigments.

   a. Urochrome is a sulfur-containing oxidation product of the colorless urochromogen. Urochromogen is oxidized to urochrome following exposure to air or by addition of one or two drops of 1% potassium permanganate (Weisz test).

   b. Urobilin is a degradation product of hemoglobin.

C. ABNORMAL URINE COLOR

Consult Table 9.

Table 9

Some Causes of Different Urine Colors

PALE YELLOW, YELLOW OR AMBER Normal urochromes and urobilin	BROWNISH Methemoglobin Melanin

DEEP YELLOW
Highly concentrated urine
Quinicrine (Atabrine);
  following acidification*
Nitrofurantoin*
Phenacetin*
Riboflavin (large quantities)*
	Salicylazosulfapyridine
	  (Azulfadine)*
	Nitrofurantoin*
	Phenacetin*
	Naphthalene*
	Sulfonamides*
	Bismuth*
	Mercury*

BLUE Methylene blue Indigo carmine and indigo blue dye* Indicans* Pseudomonas infections*	YELLOW-BROWN, GREEN-BROWN Bile pigments
GREEN (MIXTURE OF BLUE + YELLOW) Methylene blue Dithiazanine iodide (Dizan) Indigo blue* Evan's blue* Biliverdin Riboflavin* Thymol*	BROWN TO BLACK (BROWN OR REDDISH BROWN WHEN VIEWED IN BRIGHT LIGHT OR IN THIN LAYER) Melanin Methemoglobin Myoglobin Bile pigments Thymol* Phenolic Compounds (ingested or from decomposed protein)* Nitrofurantoins*
ORANGE-YELLOW Highly concentrated urine Excess urobilin Bilirubin Pyridium Phenazopyridine* Salicylazosulfapyridine (Azulfadine)* Fluorescein sodium*	Nitrites* Naphthalene* Chlorinated hydrocarbons* Analine dyes* Homogentisic acid* COLORLESS Very dilute urine
RED, PINK, RED-BROWN, RED-ORANGE, ORANGE Hematuria Hemoglobinuria Myoglobinuria (red-brown) Porphyrinuria Congo red Phenosulfonphthalein (following alkalinization) Neoprontosil Warfarin (Orange)* Rhubarb* Carbon tetrachloride* Phenazopyridine* Phenothiazines* Diphenylhydantoin*	MILKY WHITE Chyle Pus Phosphate crystals

*reported in human beings

III. ODOR

A. Normal urine has a characteristic odor which varies between species and sex. For example, the odor of urine from non-castrated male cats is strong and unmistakably characteristic.

B. Detection of abnormal urine odors indicates the need for further evaluation.

1. Detection of abnormal urine odors is rarely of specific diagnostic significance.

2. In man, abnormal urine odors in newborn infants are sometimes associated with metabolic defects and urinary tract infections.

3. Excretion of drugs, such as ampicillin, may be associated with abnormal and sometimes characteristic odors.

4. The cause of abnormal urine odor is best determined by evaluation of a complete urinalysis. Depending on the cause, additional laboratory tests and/or clinical investigation may be required.

C. AMMONIACAL (NH_3) ODORS

1. An ammoniacal odor is a common abnormality of urine.

   a. NH_3 imparts characteristic odor; NH_4^+ and urea are odorless.

b. Fresh normal urine at room temperature does not have an ammoniacal odor because it contains an insignificant quantity of NH_3. It contains large quantities of urea, however, and may contain a large quantity of NH_4^+.

2. Potential causes of ammoniacal odor include:

a. Urea which has been degraded to NH_3 by urease-producing bacteria.
(1) Urease-producing bacteria may be pathogens or contaminants.
(2) Freshly-voided urine with an ammoniacal odor suggests (but does not prove) infection of the urinary tract with urease-producing bacteria.

b. NH_4^+ transformed to NH_3 by exogenous heat.

3. A putrid odor indicates bacterial degradation of a large quantity of protein.

4. Ketonuria has been reported to impart a characteristic odor to urine.

a. Many individuals are unable to detect this odor.

b. Laboratory tests provide a more reliable index of ketonuria.

IV. TRANSPARENCY—TURBIDITY

A. In most species, freshly voided urine is transparent.
1. Concentrated urine is more likely to be turbid than dilute urine.
2. *In vitro* alterations, especially changes in temperature and pH, may cause varying degrees of loss of transparency.

B. The degree of turbidity is commonly estimated by reading newspaper print through a clear container filled with urine.

C. The cause of urine turbidity is usually best explained by evaluation of urine sediment.

D. Potential causes of urine turbidity include one or more of the following:
1. Crystals.
2. Red blood cells, white blood cells, and/or epithelial cells.
3. Semen.
4. Bacteria, yeasts, *etc.*
5. Contaminants from the collection chamber.
6. Lipids (tend to rise to surface).
7. Mucus.
8. Contamination with feces.

E. Crystals are a common cause of turbidity.
1. The solubility of most crystals is influenced by temperature. Hence, crystals may form as urine at body temperature cools to room temperature. If crystals interfere with microscopic examination of sediment, their dissolution may be prompted by warming the sample in a 37° C water bath.
2. Precipitation of crystals may also be influenced by pH. Consult Chapter 8, section on Interpretation, Crystals, urine sediment, for further information.

F. Hematuria vs. hemoglobinuria.
1. Hematuria typically results in brownish to red (occasionally black) turbid urine.
2. Hemoglobinuria (and myoglobinuria) results in brownish to red (occasionally black) transparent urine.

Chapter 6. Determination of Solute Concentration of Urine by Osmolality, Specific Gravity, and Refractive Index

Determination of Solute Concentration of Urine
by Osmolality, Specific Gravity and Refractive Index

I. INDICATIONS

There are two major indications for routine evaluation of specific gravity of all urine samples analyzed:

A. Interpretation of other results of the urinalysis is dependent on knowledge of specific gravity (or osmolality) since this data provides information regarding the ratio of solutes to solvent (water).

1. Tests of routine urinalyses are typically performed on a relatively small sample of urine without regard to the rate of formation of urine or total urine volume. Semiquantitative interpretation of results is unfeasible in such samples without knowledge of specific gravity.

2. Protein is used as an example: A 2+ proteinuria at a specific gravity of 1.010 reflects a much greater loss of protein than a 2+ proteinuria at 1.030. The same concept is applicable to interpretation of the significance of glucose, bilirubin, constituents in urine sediment, *etc.*

B. Urine specific gravity and/or osmolality is used to assess the ability of the renal tubules to concentrate (*i.e.*, remove water in excess of solute) or dilute (*i.e.*, remove solute in excess of water) glomerular filtrate. Knowledge of urine specific gravity is extremely helpful when attempting to localize azotemia (*see* Table 8).

II. METHODOLOGY

A. OSMOLALITY

1. Applied physics:

   a. Dissolution of one or more substances (or solutes) in a solvent (water) changes four mathematically interrelated physical characteristics (known as colligative properties): osmotic pressure, freezing point, vapor pressure, and boiling point. These properties are all directly related to the total number of solute particles within the solution and independent of the homogeneity or nonhomogeneity of molecular species, molecular weight and molecule size.

   b. As solute is added to solvent:
      (1) Osmotic pressure increases.
      (2) Freezing point decreases.
      (3) Vapor pressure decreases.
      (4) Boiling point increases.

   c. Changes in these colligative properties are dependent on the number of particles of solute in solution and *not* on other characteristics, such as molecular weight, electrical charge, chemical nature or shape of dissolved particles.

   d. A 1 gm/dl solution of NaCl has many hundred times the osmotic activity of a 1 gm/dl solution of plasma proteins because undissociated and dissociated salt molecules contribute many small molecules in large numbers while the same weight of protein contributes fewer large molecules in smaller numbers.

2. In clinical medicine, the osmotic concentration of solutions is usually measured with instruments that determine freezing points (freezing point osmometer) or vapor pressure (vapor pressure osmometer).

   a. Commercial osmometers determine osmolality by measuring relative changes in freezing point or vapor pressure of unknown solutions, utilizing standard solutions as reference points.

   b. Currently available equipment provides rapid digital

readout of data on samples as small as 0.2 ml.

c. Unfortunately, osmometers are relatively expensive.

d. Vapor pressure osmometers appear to be superior to freezing point osmometers for use in veterinary medicine because of the potential for measurement of extremely high solute concentrations of urine samples. In studies of concentrated feline urine performed at the University of Minnesota, freezing point osmometers were not capable of accurately measuring the osmotic concentration of samples greater than SG = 1.050.

e. Although osmometers provide a measurement of the number (or concentration) of osmotically active particles in solution, they do not indicate the type(s) of solute present.

2. Applied physiological chemistry:

a. The unit of osmotic concentration is the *osmole*.

(1) One osmole of an ideal solution in one kilogram of water will have a freezing point of $-1.86°$ C compared to pure water.

(2) Since the *osmole* represents a large mass of solute, the *milliosmole* has been developed for clinical use.

(a) One milliosmole (mOsm) = 0.001 osmole.

(b) Use of milliosmoles eliminates the necessity of using fractions when evaluating osmolality of biological fluids.

(3) For osmolality the unit of solvent measurement is mass (kg), and therefore osmolality is expressed as mOsm/kg of solution. For osmolarity the unit of solvent measurement is volume (liter), and therefore osmolarity is expressed as mOsm/L of solution. The numerical difference between osmolality and osmolarity values of biological fluids is usually small, and therefore the values are commonly used\interchangeably.

b. Osmotic activity in the body.

(1) Sodium, chloride, and bicarbonate account for approximately 90% of the osmotic activity of extracellular fluid. Nonelectrolytes, such as urea, proteins, and glucose, account for the remainder of the osmotic activity.

(2) Sodium, chloride, and urea account for the majority of osmotic activity in urine.

(3) There is usually no significant difference between the osmolality (or specific gravity) of uncentrifuged urine and the supernatant of centrifuged urine because cells, casts, *etc.*, do not contribute significantly to osmotic pressure.

(4) There is no significant difference between serum and plasma osmolality since fibrinogen does not exert a significant osmotic effect. The quantity and type of anticoagulant used to obtain plasma may be of significance, however. For example, EDTA may contribute 5 to 20 mOsm/kg to plasma osmolality, depending on the amount of blood in a 2 ml Vacutainer® tube.

(5) The osmotic concentration of plasma, serum, interstitial fluid, transcellular fluid, and intracellular fluid is approximately 300 mOsm/kg of water.

(6) Normally the osmotic concentration of urine is variable, being dependent on the fluid and electrolyte balance of the body, and the nitrogen content of the diet. Species differences in the ability to concentrate urine are also significant (*see* Table 10).

(7) The ratio of urine osmolality (U_{osm}) to plasma osmolality (P_{osm}) is a good clinical index of the ability of the kidneys to concentrate or dilute glomerular filtrate.

(a) A U/P_{osm} ratio above one indicates that the kidneys are concentrating urine above plasma and glomerular filtrate. Following water deprivation, the U/P_{osm} of normal dogs may be 7 or higher.

(b) A U/P_{osm} ratio of approximately one indicates that water and solute are being excreted in a state that is iso-osmotic with plasma.

(c) A U/P_{osm} ratio significantly below one indicates that the tubules are capable of absorbing solute in excess of water (*i.e.*, they are diluting glomerular filtrate).

B. SPECIFIC GRAVITY

1. DEFINITION AND CHARACTERISTICS:

a. Urine specific gravity is a measurement of the density of urine compared to pure water. Stated in another way, urine specific gravity is the ratio of the weight of urine to the weight of an equal volume of water, both measured at the same temperature $\left(SG = \frac{\text{wt. of urine}}{\text{wt. of water}}\right)$.

(1) The SG of water is 1.000.

(2) Urine is more dense than water because it is composed of water and various solutes of different densities.

b. There is only an approximate relationship between specific gravity and total solute concentration. In addition to the number of molecules of solute, SG is influenced by other factors including molecular size and molecular weight of solutes. Each species of solute has its own characteristic effect on the SG of urine.

(1) Urine samples having equivalent numbers of solute molecules *per* unit volume may have different SG values if different mixtures of solutes are present.

(2) Equal numbers of molecules of urea, sodium chloride, albumin, globulin, fibrinogen, and glucose all have a different quantitative effect on specific gravity.

(3) Addition of either of the following substances to 100 ml of urine will increase SG by 0.001:

(a) 0.147 grams of sodium chloride.

(b) 0.36 grams of urea.

(c) 0.27 grams of glucose.

(d) 0.4 grams of albumin.

c. Urine SG is affected by temperature.

(1) Although the weight of urine remains constant regardless of its temperature, the density of urine decreases with an increase in temperature. Conversely, the density of urine increases with a decrease in temperature.

(2) For precise work, the temperature of urine should be compared with the reference temperature of the instrument used to determine SG (*see* Figure 13).

d. Urine SG is a direct, but not proportional, function of the number of solute particles in urine.

(1) Urine SG varies with the kind of solute present, whereas urine osmolality is independent of the types of solute present.

(2) Urine specific gravity provides only an estimation of osmolality. It is useful as a screening procedure, but may be unsuitable in some circumstances requiring more precise evaluation of renal tubular concentration and diluting capacity.

2. METHODOLOGY—URINOMETERS

a. A urinometer is a type of hydrometer consisting of a weighted bulb attached to a graduated cylindrical stem. A scale etched on the surface or placed inside the stem is calibrated in specific gravity units.

b. Urinometers are calibrated at a reference temperature (usually close to room temperature). The reference temperature is usually identified on the stem (Figure 13). For precise work, measurements should be corrected by adding 0.001 for each 3° C that urine temperature is above the reference temperature of the urinometer, or by subtracting 0.001 for each 3° C that urine temperature is below the reference temperature. For screening evaluation, this calculation is unnecessary, although the concept should be considered when interpreting the results.

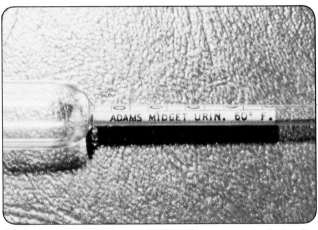

Fig. 13. Photograph of midget urinometer. Note reference temperature in stem. The paper scale within the stem could significantly alter results if it is moved.

c. The precision of urinometers is not great.

(1) Measurements vary with temperature.

(2) There may be difficulty in reading the meniscus. Froth or bubbles on the surface of urine should be broken (touch with a piece of filter paper), and the reading taken at the level of the bottom of the meniscus.

(3) There is a tendency for urinometers to "drag" against the side of narrow deep cylinders containing the urine sample. This even may induce erroneous values.

(4) The specific gravity scales of urinometers are often inaccurate. Each urinometer should be checked for accuracy after purchase and periodically thereafter.

(a) Distilled water has an SG = 1.000.

(b) 17.39 gms of $CuSO_4 \cdot 5H_2O/L$ has an SG = 1.010; 65.07 gms of $CuSO_4 \cdot 5H_2O/L$ has an SG = 1.040.

(c) 75 ml of xylene and 28 ml of bromobenzene have an SG = 1.030.

d. Determination of urine specific gravity with a urinometer requires a relatively large sample of urine (*i.e.*, 5 to 15 ml or more depending on the size of the urinometer and the size of the container). Specific gravity may be determined on small samples of urine by addition of a known volume of water and by correcting the observed measurement for the dilution.

(1) To obtain the actual specific gravity of a diluted urine sample, to the value 1.000 add the product obtained when the observed value minus 1.000 is multiplied by the dilution factor. For example, if the dilution is one part urine to two parts water, and the observed specific gravity is 1.007, the corrected specific gravity is 1.021 (1.007 minus 1.000 = 0.007; 0.007 x 3 = 0.021; 1 + 0.021 = 1.021).

(2) Values obtained by the dilution method are less accurate than undiluted values because of the error introduced by measurement, and because the reading error is multiplied by the dilution factor.

C. REFRACTIVE INDEX

1. DEFINITION AND CHARACTERISTICS:

a. Refractive index is defined as the ratio of the velocity of light in the air to the velocity of light in a solution. Aqueous solutions such as urine contain substances which absorb various wavelengths of light, and as a consequence "bend" light rays. The degree of "bending" may be measured by an instrument called a refractometer.

b. Like specific gravity, the refractive index of urine is related to the quantity of solutes present, and to the characteristics of the solutes present. It therefore provides an estimate of osmotic concentration.

2. METHODOLOGY—REFRACTOMETERS:

a. Small hand-held refractometers, calibrated to determine urine specific gravity, are available. The instru-

ments may also be calibrated to provide results in terms of refractive index or total solids.

b. There is considerable variability in the quality and cost of refractometers. We have the greatest confidence in the Goldberg refractometer, since it typically provides reproducible results, has an adjustable scale, and contains a built-in mechanism for temperature correction (from 60 to 100° F). Improvements in newer models have also increased reproducibility of results (*see* Appendix).

c. Refractometers are calibrated at a reference temperature. Within limits, however, their design permits temperature compensation.

(1) Because the temperature of the small drop of urine required to obtain a measurement with refractometers rapidly equilibrates with temperature of the instrument, a temperature-corrected result may be obtained, provided the instrument's temperature is near the reference temperature. Caution should be used to prevent significant alterations in the temperature of the instrument by holding it for prolonged periods, storing it adjacent to heating vents, *etc.*

(2) Goldberg refractometers and some other models have a built-in temperature compensating mechanism.

D. OSMOMETERS VERSUS REFRACTOMETERS VERSUS URINOMETERS

1. Osmometers provide a more accurate assessment of osmolality of individual urine samples than refractometers or urinometers, and therefore should be used when errors in the assessment of renal function are of significant consequence (*i.e.*, in conjunction with water deprivation and vasopressin response tests).

2. Refractometry is entirely satisfactory for routine screening by urinalysis.

3. Refractometers are recommended over urinometers for determination of urine specific gravity because:
   a. They provide more reproducible results.
   b. They require a small sample size.
   c. They are temperature-compensated.
   d. They are technically easy to use.

III. INTERPRETATION

A. NORMAL (Table 10)

Table 10

Osmolality and Specific Gravity Values for Adult Dog, Cat and Human Urine

	SPECIES		
Factor	Dog	Cat	Human
Range of Normal SG	1.001-±1.065	1.001-±1.080	1.001-±1.035
Usual SG— Normal hydration	1.015–1.045	1.035–1.060	1.015–1.025
Range of Normal osmolality (mOsm/kg)	50 to 2500	50 to 3000+	50 to 1500

1. The SG of urine of normal dogs and cats is variable, being dependent on the fluid and electrolyte balance of the body, the nitrogen content of the diet, and other variables related to species and individuals. The urine SG often fluctuates widely from day to day and within the same day.

2. Urine specific gravity may range from 1.001 to 1.065 or greater in adult normal dogs, and from 1.001 to 1.080 or greater in adult normal cats. Depending on the requirements of the body for water and/or solutes, any specific gravity value within these ranges may be normal. Therefore, the concept of an average normal specific gravity is misleading, because it implies that values above or below the average may not be normal.

3. Randomly collected urine samples from normal adult dogs and cats often have a specific gravity that encompasses a narrower range than that just mentioned (approximately 1.015 to 1.045 for dogs, and 1.035 to 1.060 for cats) (see Table 10), but an individual urine sample with a specific gravity outside these values is not reliable evidence of renal dysfunction.

4. Maximum, minimum, and typical specific gravity values for infant and immature dogs and cats have apparently not been evaluated. In newborn infants, the kidneys can only concentrate urine to about 1½ to 2 times plasma osmolality. The time of maturation of various renal functions in immature dogs and cats is unknown. Appropriate caution must be used when interpreting the significance of urine specific gravity and osmolality values in immature animals since they may not be the same as those commonly used for adult animals.

5. A urine specific gravity which is similar to that of glomerular filtrate (1.008 to 1.012) may be observed in individuals with normal renal function, since the ability of normal kidneys to influence specific gravity encompasses these values. Since such values may be normal or abnormal, they should be viewed as presumptive evidence of an abnormality. Further data will be required, however, to prove or disprove this presumption.

6. The ability of patients to excrete urine with a specific gravity significantly above that of glomerular filtrate (1.008 to 1.012) is dependent on an intact system for production and release of antidiuretic hormone, a sufficient population of functional nephrons to generate and maintain a high solute concentration in the renal medulla, and a sufficient population of functional tubules to respond to antidiuretic hormone.

   a. Data obtained from experimental studies in dogs suggest that only about one-third of the nephrons of both kidneys are required to concentrate urine to 1.025 or greater. Stated in another way, significant impairment of the kidneys' ability to concentrate (or dilute) urine is usually not detected until at least two-thirds of the total renal functional parenchyma has been impaired. In general, patients with at least one-third of the total nephron population functional have adequate renal function to prevent clinical signs of primary renal failure. Consult Chapter 1, DEFINITIONS OF TERMS AND CONCEPTS, for additional information pertaining to renal disease and renal failure.

   b. The minimum quantity of functional nephrons required to concentrate urine to a specific gravity of 1.025 in human beings and cats has apparently not been determined. Because of significant interspecies differences in the ability to maximally concentrate urine (see Table 10), it seems logical to assume that the number would be different from that in dogs. Further studies are required before meaningful generalities can be established.

7. Significane of Urine SG of 1.025 in man, dogs and cats.

   a. The ability of dogs to concentrate urine to a specific gravity of 1.025 has been generally accepted as evidence of "adequate" renal concentrating capacity (i.e., at least one-third of the total nephron population is functional) to maintain homeostasis.

   b. It appears that the urine specific gravity end point of

Figure 14

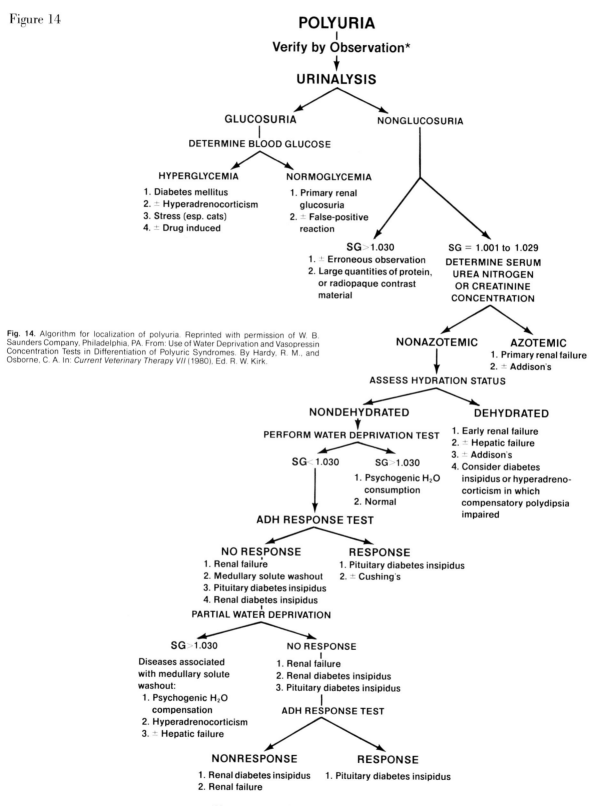

Fig. 14. Algorithm for localization of polyuria. Reprinted with permission of W. B. Saunders Company, Philadelphia, PA. From: Use of Water Deprivation and Vasopressin Concentration Tests in Differentiation of Polyuric Syndromes. By Hardy, R. M., and Osborne, C. A. In: *Current Veterinary Therapy VII* (1980), Ed. R. W. Kirk.

1.025 used by many veterinarians has been extrapolated from human data. Since human beings can concentrate their urine to a maximum of 1.035 to 1.040, whereas values for dogs may reach 1.060 or more, and values for cats may reach 1.080 or more, concentration of urine to 1.025 probably implies better renal tubular function in man than in cats or dogs.

c. Uncontrolled clinical observations in dogs indicate that detection of a urine specific gravity ≥ 1.025 indicates an adequate population of nephrons to prevent clinical signs associated with primary renal failure.
   (1) A significant degree of renal disease may exist in dogs able to concentrate their urine to a specific gravity of 1.025.
   (2) In one study, the maximal urine specific gravities of three partially nephrectomized dogs (two-thirds of total nephrons removed) subjected to 48 hours of water deprivation were 1.023, 1.018 and 1.027.

d. Experimental studies recently performed on cats at the University of Georgia revealed that animals with less than 25% functional nephrons could concentrate their urine significantly higher than SG=1.025. Further studies in cats are required to determine the urine SG value that indicates an adequate population of functional nephrons to prevent clinical signs associated with primary renal failure.

8. Since metabolic work is required to dilute glomerular filtrate (SG = 1.008 to 1.012) by removing solute in excess of water, a urine SG significantly below 1.008 indicates that a sufficient number of functional nephrons (commonly estimated to be at least one-third of the total population) are present to prevent clinical signs associated with primary renal failure.

B. ABNORMAL

1. Consult Chapter 1, DEFINITIONS OF TERMS AND CONCEPTS, for information related to renal disease, renal failure and uremia.
2. Interpretation of urine SG values of randomly obtained samples is dependent on knowledge of the patient's hydration status, the plasma or serum concentration of urea nitrogen or creatinine, and knowledge of drugs or fluids that have been administered to the patient. Knowledge of urine volume and water consumption may also be helpful. In some instances, interpretation may require knowledge of urine and plasma osmolality.
3. Consult Chapter 5, PHYSICAL PROPERTIES OF URINE, section on urine volume, for additional information related to physiologic and pathologic polyuria, and physiologic and pathologic oliguria. Knowledge of urine SG (or osmolality) is of great value in localizing the source of abnormal urine volume (Figure 14).
4. Varying degrees of impaired ability to concentrate or dilute glomerular filtrate are a consistent finding in all forms of primary renal failure.
   a. Because the kidneys have tremendous reserve capacity, impairment of their ability to concentrate or dilute urine may not be detected until at least two-thirds (dogs) or more (cats) of the total population of nephrons has been damaged.
   b. Complete inability of the nephrons to modify glomerular filtrate typically results in formation of urine with a specific gravity which is similar to that of glomerular filtrate (1.008 to 1.012). This phenomenon has been commonly called "fixation of specific gravity."
   c. Total loss of the ability to concentrate and dilute urine (SG = 1.008 to 1.012) often does not occur as a sudden event, but may develop gradually. For this reason urine specific gravity values of approximately 1.007 to 1.029 in dogs, and 1.007 to 1.034 in cats associated with clinical dehydration and/or azotemia are highly suggestive of primary renal failure.
   d. Contrary to statements widely publicized at one time, acute renal diseases of sufficient severity to cause primary renal failure are not associated with marked elevation in urine specific gravity values. Azotemia associated with hypersthenuria should prompt a high index of suspicion of prerenal azotemia.
   e. Once the urine specific gravity reflects impaired ability to concentrate or dilute urine (1.007 to ± 1.029 in dogs), it is more an index of nephron function than of distal tubular and collecting duct function since, in addition to generalized tubular lesions, this abnormality may occur as a result of factors not specifically related to tubular damage. These factors include:
   (1) Compensatory increase in glomerular filtration which occurs as a result of a decrease in the quantity of functional nephrons. Increased production of glomerular filtrate floods the distal tubules and collecting ducts. It is associated with

CHAPTER 6

decreased fractional tubular reabsorption of sodium and phosphorus by viable nephrons.

(2) Decrease in the number of functioning nephrons. The latter is associated with impaired ability to maintain the high osmotic gradient normally present in renal medulla.

(3) Increased glomerular filtration of solutes retained in plasma (urea, creatinine, phosphorus, *etc.*) which induce an osmotic diuresis. This accentuates the degree of obligatory polyuria.

f. Once the ability to concentrate or dilute urine has been permanently destroyed, repeated evaluation of specific gravity will not be of aid in evaluation of progressive deterioration of renal function. Therefore, serial evaluation of urine specific gravity is of greatest aid in detecting functional changes earlier during the course of primary renal failure, or in monitoring functional recovery associated with reversible renal diseases.

g. If sufficient clinical evidence is present to warrant examination of the patient's renal function by determining the serum concentration of creatinine or blood urea nitrogen, the urine specific gravity (or osmolality) should be evaluated at the same time.

(1) As emphasized in the previous discussion, a concentrated urine sample associated with an abnormal elevation in serum creatinine or urea nitrogen concentration suggests the probability of *prerenal azotemia.*

(2) If nonazotemic patients have impaired ability to concentrate urine, causes of pathologic polyuria should be explored. Determination of urine specific gravity or osmolality may allow one to determine whether a disorder characterized by water (1.001 to ± 1.006) or solute (± 1.008 or greater) diuresis is probable. Consult section on urine volume, Chapter 5, PHYSICAL PROPERTIES OF URINE, for additional information.

(3) Azotemia associated with a specific gravity of 1.007 to ± 1.029 (dogs) or ± 1.034 (cats) indicates the probability of primary renal failure, although on occasion hypoadrenocorticism may induce similar findings.

(4) If a *nondehydrated, nonazotemic* patient suspected of having pathologic polyuria does not have a

urine specific gravity which indicates that the kidneys can definitely concentrate urine, further tests are required before any meaningful conclusions can be established about the kidneys' capacity to concentrate urine.

(a) When the patient is deprived of water for an appropriate period of time, antidiuretic hormone will normally be released from the posterior pituitary gland as a compensatory response to hydropenia. Antidiuretic hormone enhances fluid reabsorption from the distal tubules and collecting ducts by increasing tubular cell permeability to water.

(1) Clinical experience has revealed that the results of water deprivation tests are often difficult to reproduce. Boundary values have been established, above which renal function is assumed to be adequate, and below which it is assumed to be impaired. A zone of doubt exists in between.

(2) Uncontrolled clinical observations indicate that dogs with "adequate" renal function will excrete urine with a high specific gravity (≥ 1.030), high osmolality, and relatively small volume (physiologic oliguria).

(3) Studies of dogs with completely normal renal function were interpreted to indicate that 95% of normal dogs subjected to water deprivation sufficient to produce a slight degree of dehydration should have a urine specific gravity of at least 1.048, a urine osmolality of at least 1,787 mOsm/kg, and a U/P$_{osm}$ ratio of at least 5.7:1. If such values are not obtained, nephron dysfunction may exist. The degree of dysfunction, however, may not be severe enough to be associated with clinical signs.

(b) Patients unable to concentrate urine following appropriately conducted water deprivation tests should be evaluated for diseases that cause medullary solute washout, and/or pituitary diabetes insipidus.

5. Urine specific gravity and localization of azotemia (*see* Table 8).

a. Although the following generalities apply to dogs and

50

cats, it is emphasized that azotemic cats with primary renal failure may be able to concentrate their urine to an SG>1.025.

(1) In dogs with primary renal failure, azotemia usually follows loss of the ability to concentrate urine to this degree.

(2) In cats with primary renal failure, azotemia may precede loss of the ability to concentrate urine to this degree.

(3) Pending further studies, we have defined SG = 1.030 as indicative of adequate urine concentration in dogs. A comparable SG value in cats is 1.035.

b. Prerenal azotemia.

(1) Pathogenesis and causes:

(a) Extraurinary diseases may cause varying degrees of alteration in glomerular filtration as a result of reduction of renal blood flow. Inadequate perfusion of normal glomeruli with blood, regardless of cause (dehydration, cardiac diseases, shock, hypoadrenocorticism, decreased plasma colloidal osmotic pressure) may cause prerenal azotemia (see Table 2).

(b) Prerenal azotemia is initially associated with structurally normal kidneys which are capable of quantitatively normal renal function, provided compromised renal perfusion is corrected prior to the onset of ischemic nephron damage. Development of primary renal failure due to ischemia prolongs and reduces the likelihood of complete recovery.

(c) In dogs, a diagnosis of prerenal azotemia should be considered if abnormal elevation in the serum or plasma concentration of urea nitrogen and creatinine is associated with concentrated urine (specific gravity ≥ 1.030) in patients with no specific evidence of generalized glomerular disease. The same generality applies to cats with a urine specific gravity ≥ 1.035.

(1) Detection of a urine specific gravity greater than approximately 1.030 in association with azotemia indicates that a sufficient quantity of functional nephrons are present to concentrate urine (i.e., at least one-third of the total nephron population).

(2) Significant elevations in the serum or plasma

concentration of urea nitrogen or creatinine due to primary renal failure cannot be detected in dogs until approximately 70 to 75% of the nephron population is nonfunctional.

(3) Elevation in urine specific gravity associated with prerenal azotemia probably reflects a compensatory response by the body to combat low perfusion pressure and blood volume by secreting antidiuretic hormone (and possibly other substances) to conserve water filtered through the glomeruli.

(4) Restoration of renal perfusion by appropriate volume replacement therapy is typically followed by a dramatic drop in the concentration of serum urea nitrogen and creatinine to normal in approximately one to three days.

(d) Another form of potentially reversible prerenal azotemia may develop in glomerulonephritic patients with severe hypoproteinemia. Although reduction in colloidal osmotic pressure as a consequence of hypoalbuminemia tends to enhance glomerular filtration rate at the level of glomeruli, this effect is usually minimized by a reduction in systemic vascular volume as a consequence of hypoalbuminemia. The net effect of severe hypoalbuminemia, therefore, is usually reduction on glomerular filtration. This may result in a proportionate degree of retention of substances normally cleared by the kidneys (creatinine, urea, etc.) (see Table 2).

(1) Therefore, the significance of abnormal increase in the serum concentration of urea nitrogen or creatinine (or a reduction in creatinine clearance) must be carefully defined in hypoproteinemic nephrotic patients.

(2) Azotemia cannot be accepted as indisputable evidence of severe primary glomerular lesions since it may be associated with a potentially reversible decrease in renal perfusion caused by hypoalbuminemia.

2. Diagnosis:

(a) Elevation in BUN or creatinine concentration.

(b) Oliguria.

(c) High specific gravity (≥ 1.030 in dogs; ≥ 1.035 in cats) or osmolality.

(d) Detection of underlying cause.

(e) Dramatic correction of azotemia following administration of appropriate therapy to restore renal perfusion.

3. Prognosis:

(a) Dependent on reversibility of primary cause.

(b) Favorable for renal function if perfusion rapidly restored.

(c) *Complete* loss of renal perfusion in excess of two to four hours will result in generalized ischemic renal disease. With the exception of shock, this degree of reduced renal perfusion is uncommon. Thus, the onset of generalized renal disease would be expected to require a longer period of altered renal perfusion.

c. Postrenal azotemia.

(1) Pathogenesis:

(a) Diseases which prevent excretion of urine from the body may cause postrenal azotemia.

(b) Initially, the kidneys are structurally normal and capable of quantitatively normal function provided the underlying cause is corrected.

(c) If the underlying cause is allowed to persist, death from alterations in water, electrolyte and acid-base and endocrine balance, in addition to accumulation of metabolic waste products, will occur within a few days. If partial obstruction to urine outflow allows the patient to survive for a longer time, varying degrees of hydronephrosis may also occur.

(2) Causes:

(a) Complete obstruction of urine outflow (*i.e.*, obstruction in urethra, bladder, or both ureters) which persists for more than 24 hours usually results in postrenal azotemia.

(b) Unilateral ureteral occlusion (an example of renal disease) is not associated with azotemia unless generalized disease of the nonobstructed kidney is also present. Consult Chapter 1, **DEFINITIONS OF TERMS AND CONCEPTS**, section on Terms and Concepts Related to Renal Disease, Renal Failure, and Uremia.

(c) Azotemia, which occurs as a sequela to rupture of the excretory pathway (most commonly the bladder), is primarily related to absorption of urine from the peritoneal cavity. Unless damaged as a result of hypovolemic shock or trauma secondary to the underlying cause of rupture of the excretory pathway, the kidneys are structurally normal.

(3) Diagnosis:

(a) Obstructive lesions.

(1) Elevation in serum urea nitrogen or creatinine concentration.

(2) Oliguria or anuria, dysuria, tenesmus.

(3) Detection of obstructive lesion(s) by physical examination (urethral plug, herniated bladder, *etc.*), radiography, *etc.*

(b) Rupture in excretory pathway.

(1) Elevation in serum urea nitrogen or creatinine concentration.

(2) Severe depression, painful abdomen, ascites.

(3) History of trauma.

(4) Inability to palpate bladder.

(5) Paracentesis (modified transudate or exudate).

(6) Retrograde contrast (positive or negative) cystography or urethrocystography.

(c) Because of its variability, the urine specific gravity of patients with postrenal azotemia is not relied on to the same degree for assessment of renal function as it is in patients with primary renal and prerenal azotemia.

(4) Prognosis:

(a) Obstructive lesions.

(1) If the patient has total obstruction to urine outflow for a period of three to six days, death from uremia will occur. Death usually occurs before significant structural changes caused by obstruction have time to develop (*i.e.*, hydronephrosis). Death is caused by alteration of fluid, acid-base, electrolyte, nutrient and endocrine balances, and accumulation of metabolic waste products.

(2) The prognosis is favorable for renal function if the obstructive lesion(s) is rapidly removed.

(3) The long-term prognosis is dependent on the reversibility of the underlying cause.

(b) Rupture of excretory pathway.

(1) Death from uremia usually occurs if the rent is not rapidly repaired.

(2) The prognosis is favorable for renal function if the rent is rapidly repaired.

(3) Long-term prognosis is dependent on the reversibility of the underlying cause.

d. Primary renal azotemia.

(1) Pathogenesis:

(a) Primary renal failure may be caused by a large number of disease processes which have in common destruction of approximately three-fourths or more of the parenchyma of both kidneys.

(b) Depending on the biological behavior of the disease in question, primary renal failure may be reversible or irreversible, acute or chronic.

(2) Diagnosis:

(a) In dogs, impairment of at least two-thirds of the nephron mass is indicated if a dehydrated patient (that has not received fluid therapy) has impaired ability to concentrate urine (SG = 1.007 to 1.029).

(1) Total loss of ability to concentrate and dilute urine does not always occur as a sudden event, but often develops gradually. For this reason a urine specific gravity between approximately 1.007 to 1.029 associated with clinical dehydration or azotemia is indicative of primary renal azotemia (see Table 8).

(2) Total inability of the nephrons to concentrate or dilute urine (so-called fixation of specific gravity or isosthenuria) results in the formation of urine that is similar to that of glomerular filtrate (approximately 1.008 to 1.012).

(b) Impairment of at least three-fourths of the functional capacity of the nephron mass is indicated if a patient has an elevation in the serum or plasma concentration of urea nitrogen and creatinine and impaired ability to concentrate or dilute urine.

(c) More definitive studies (biopsy, radiography, exploratory surgery, etc.) are required to establish the underlying cause of primary renal failure.

(d) Remember, uremic signs are not directly caused by renal lesions, but rather are related to varying degrees of fluid, acid-base, electrolyte and nutrient imbalances, vitamin and endocrine alterations, and retention of waste products of protein catabolism, which develop as a result of damage to nephrons.

e. Glomerulotubular imbalance.

(1) Abnormal elevation in the serum concentration of urea nitrogen or creatinine may occur in association with an elevated urine specific gravity in some patients with primary renal failure caused by generalized renal disease.

(a) Caution should be used not to overinterpret the absolute value of the urine specific gravity in such patients, since it may be falsely elevated by the effect of protein.

(b) Addition of 400 mg of protein per 100 ml of urine will increase the urine specific gravity by approximately 0.001.

(2) The renal lesion in such patients must be characterized by glomerular damage which is sufficiently severe to impair renal clearance of urea and creatinine, but which has not yet induced a sufficient degree of ischemic atrophy and necrosis of renal tubular cells to prevent urine concentration. Thus glomerular filtrate that is formed can be concentrated, at least to some degree.

(3) This group of patients may be differentiated from patients with prerenal azotemia by failure of a search for one of the extrarenal causes of poor perfusion, by the presence of persistent proteinuria, and by lack of response to restoration of vascular volume and perfusion with appropriate therapy (Table 11).

Table 11
Differentiation of Prerenal Azotemia from Primary Azotemia Associated with Glomerulotubular Imbalance

FACTOR	PRERENAL AZOTEMIA	GLOMERULOTUBULAR IMBALANCE AND PRIMARY RENAL AZOTEMIA
BUN	Increased	Increased
Creatinine	Increased	Increased
Urine specific gravity	≥ 1.030	1.015−1.025
Proteinuria	Usually negative	Positive
Prerenal cause	Present	Absent
Response to correction of renal perfusion	Within 1-3 days	Minimal

f. Primary renal azotemia plus prerenal or postrenal azotemia.

(1) Pathogenesis:

(a) Severely diseased kidneys have impaired ability to compensate for stresses imposed by disease states, dietary indiscretions, changes in environment, *etc.*

(b) Uremic crises may be precipitated in patients with previously compensated primary renal disease by a variety of concomitant extrarenal factors.

(c) Postulated mechanisms of "acute on chronic" (also called "reversible on irreversible") uremic crises include the following:

(1) Factors (anorexia, infection, extensive tissue necrosis, administration of catabolic drugs) which accelerate endogenous protein catabolism increase the quantity of metabolic by-products in the body since the kidneys are incapable of excreting them. Protein by-products contribute significantly to the production of uremic signs in patients with renal failure.

(2) Stress states (fever, infection, change of environment) are associated with release of glucocorticoids from the adrenal glands. Glucocorticoids stimulate conversion of proteins to carbohydrates (gluconeogenesis) and thus increase the quantity of protein waste products in the body.

(3) Abnormalities which decrease renal perfusion (i.e., decreased water consumption, vomiting, diarrhea, shock, cardiac decompensation) cause prerenal uremia.

(4) Administration of nephrotoxic drugs may precipitate a uremic crisis by damaging nephrons.

(2) Diagnostic considerations include:

(a) Previous history of compensated primary renal failure.

(b) Detection of primary extrarenal disease processes in addition to generalized renal disease.

(c) Response to therapy, or amelioration of signs because prerenal or postrenal causes are self-limiting. Whereas patients with uremic crises precipitated by reversible extrarenal disorders (pancreatitis, hepatic disease, gastroenteritis, *etc.*) may rapidly respond to supportive and symptomatic therapy, patients with uremic crises caused by progressive irreversible destruction of nephrons will not.

Chapter 7. Chemical Characteristics

Chemical Characteristics

I. URINE pH

A. INDICATIONS

1. DIAGNOSTIC

a. Urine pH may be used as a crude index of body acid base balance.

(1) The body generally produces an excess of acid metabolites. The lungs regulate acid-base balance by retention or elimination of carbon dioxide (and, therefore, carbonic acid), while the kidneys regulate acid-base balance primarily *via* excretion of bicarbonate, ammonium ion, and phosphates.

(2) There may be significant diurnal variation in urine pH. Diet and disease may also induce considerable variation in urine pH. As was the situation with urine specific gravity, differentiation between normal and abnormal (or inappropriate) urine pH values is not possible without additional information. Both may fall within the same range.

b. Knowledge of urine pH may aid in determination of the type of uroliths present prior to their mineral analysis.

(1) Calcium phosphate (apatite) and magnesium ammonium phosphate (struvite) uroliths tend to form in alkaline urine.

(2) Cystine and uric acid uroliths tend to form in acid urine.

(3) Ammonium urate crystals may be flocculated by hydrogen ion (acid pH) or ammonium ion (alkaline pH).

(4) Formation of calcium oxalate and silica uroliths is apparently not significantly influenced by urine pH.

c. Urinary tract infections caused by urease-producing bacteria (primarily *Staphylococci* and *Proteus* spp) frequently cause urine to become alkaline. Urinary tract infections are also commonly associated with acid urine since most bacterial pathogens do not produce urease.

d. Knowledge of urine pH may be important in interpretation of findings in urine sediment. Red blood cells, white cells, casts, and other proteinaceous structures tend to disintegrate in alkaline urine.

2. THERAPEUTIC

a. Urine pH is commonly manipulated to dissolve or prevent recurrence of certain uroliths.

(1) Calcium phosphate and magnesium ammonium phosphate crystals are more soluble in acid urine.

(2) Cystine and uric acid crystals are more soluble in alkaline urine.

(3) Ammonium urate crystals are least likely to precipitate in urine without a neutral pH.

b. Because acid urine inhibits bacterial growth, urinary acidifiers are sometimes used as ancillary treatment of urinary tract infections.

c. The therapeutic efficacy of some antimicrobial agents may be enhanced by alteration of urine pH. The solubility of some antimicrobial agents may also be pH-dependent.

d. Knowledge of urine pH is commonly used as a crude index of therapeutic response when attempting to correct states of systemic acidosis or alkalosis.

e. Therapeutic manipulation of pH is also recommended in management of myoglobinuria.

B. METHODOLOGY

1. pH METERS

a. pH meters provide excellent results, but are not commonly used for routine urinalyses because they are expensive, and because of the technical ease provided by reagent strips.

b. pH meters may be used in conjunction with determination of titratable acidity. Some procedures for measurement of titratable acidity include concurrent determination of bicarbonate and ammonium ion concentration.

(1) Hydrogen ions may be excreted in urine in a form (such as monobasic phosphate or H_2PO_4) not detectable by simple pH measurements.

(2) An estimation of the amount of excess acid excreted in urine (or the amount of acid conserved in states of deficiency) during a 24-hour period as measured by titration of urine to pH 7.4 may be defined as titratable acidity.

   (a) Conceptually, titratable acidity is measured by titrating a representative aliquot of a 24-hour urine specimen with 0.1 N sodium hydroxide or hydrochloric acid to a pH of 7.4 as indicated by a pH meter.

   (b) Titratable acidity is usually reported as the number of milliliters of 0.1 NaOH or HCl required to neutralize a 24-hour specimen. It is reported as a negative or positive value depending on the quantity of HCl(−) or NaOH (+) needed to adjust the pH of urine to 7.4. A negative result indicates conservation of hydrogen ion, while a positive result indicates excretion of excess acid.

(3) Titratable acidity is primarily influenced by filtered phosphate, bicarbonate and ammonia.

(4) Diets also influence titratable acidity.

   (a) Diets rich in sulfur-containing amino acid (methionine and cystine) result in production of acid urine, because oxidation of neutral sulfate results in generation of hydrogen ion and sulfate ion.

   (b) Diets high in vegetables and fruits usually contain an excess of free anions (such as lactate, citrate, malate, *etc.*) which fix the hydrogen ion when they are catabolized to carbon dioxide and water. Thus, they tend to alkalinize urine.

(5) Proteinuria will cause a varying degree of interference with titratable acidity because of the buffering capacity of proteins.

(6) Increased production of β-hydroxybutyric acid and acetoacetic acid in ketotic states may also result in positive values for titratable acidity. The pk[1] of β-hydroxybutyric acid is 4.4. Therefore, at lower limits of urine acidification, about one-half of the β-hydroxybutyric acid will be excreted in dissociated form. The pk of acetoacetic acid is even lower, accounting for the fact that only a small amount will be excreted as free acid.

2. REAGENT STRIPS

a. Urine pH can readily be determined by any one of a number of commercially-available test strips impregnated with indicator dyes. The most reliable results are obtained by evaluation of fresh specimens.

b. Litmus paper is too insensitive for diagnostic use.

c. Nitrazine paper is capable of detecting changes in pH from 4.5 to 7.5.

   (1) The color ranges from yellow to blue and can be matched to standard colors for estimation of urine pH.

   (2) This range is too narrow for diagnostic use.

d. Wide-range hydrogen paper (pH 5.5 to 9) is satisfactory for routine analyses. It is available as LoBuff® pH Paper (*see* Appendix: Microessential Labs Inc.).

e. Diagnostic strips (Multistix®, *etc.*, Chemstrip®, *etc.*) (*see* Appendix: Ames Co.; Bio-Dynamics Inc.) contain methyl red and bromthymol blue, and are capable of monitoring changes in urine pH from 5 to 9.

   (1) Methyl red turns red in acid urine and yellow in neutral or alkaline urine.

   (2) Bromthymol blue turns green and blue in alkaline urine, and yellow in acid urine.

   (3) Care must be taken with Multistix® to prevent the buffer in the adjacent protein test from being transported by urine to the pH test pad, since this phenomenon will result in an acid pH change in a portion or all of the test pad.

C. INTERPRETATION

1. NORMAL

a. The kidneys are capable of adjusting the pH of urine between 4.5 and approximately 8.5, depending on the acid-base status of the body. Therefore, the pH of urine provides a reflection of the metabolic state of the body.

   (1) Ingestion of animal protein diets typically result in production of acid urine. The urine pH of dog and cat urine commonly lies between 5.5 and 7.0. In a study of 649 cats at the University of Minnesota, the mean urine pH was 6.6 (range 5.0 to 9.0).

   (2) Ingestion of diets primarily composed of vegetables

and cereals typically results in production of alkaline urine.

b. Urine pH tends to vary throughout the day, in part because of events associated with eating and digestion.

(1) Urine of dogs and cats tends to become less acidic shortly following ingestion of food. This is related to the "alkaline tide," and presumably is due to increased secretion of hydrochloric acid in the stomach.

(2) In one experimental study in cats fed a canned diet (C/D® Prescription Diet®), urine pH increased from a value of 6 to 7.2 within four hours after feeding.

(3) It is logical to assume that the magnitude of change in urine pH following eating will be dependent on the composition of the diet, the frequency of eating and the quantity of food consumed.

c. In man, the pH of urine obtained following sleep for several hours tends to be more acid, presumably a reflection of respiratory acidosis associated with decreased ventilation during sleep.

2. ABNORMAL (inappropriate)

a. Abnormal or inappropriate urine pH values are similar to normal values. Meaningful interpretation may require knowledge of blood pH and PCO_2, plasma bicarbonate concentration, and response to controlled administration of acidifying or alkalinizing substances.

b. The infrequency with which urine pH values below 5.5 and above 7.5 occur in dogs should arouse suspicion of an abnormality when they are observed.

c. The tendency to excrete acid urine may be associated with several disorders, including:

(1) Respiratory and metabolic acidosis.
(2) Diabetic ketoacidosis.
(3) Primary renal failure.
(4) Severe vomiting (so-called paradoxical aciduria of vomiting).
(5) Severe diarrhea.
(6) Starvation.

(7) Pyrexia.
(8) Catabolism of endogenous or exogenous proteins.
(9) Oxygen debt.

d. The tendency to excrete alkaline urine may be associated with several disorders, including:

(1) Urinary tract infections caused by urease-producing pathogens.
(2) Respiratory or metabolic alkalosis.
(3) Vomiting.
(4) Renal tubular acidosis. (More appropriately stated as an inability to acidify urine in response to body needs. The urine pH may be 6.5 or higher.)

e. Drugs which acidify urine include:

(1) Phosphate salts (sodium, potassium, or ammonium).
(2) d,l-methionine.
(3) Ammonium chloride.
(4) Ascorbic acid (although recent studies in man and cats indicate that ascorbic acid was incapable of altering urine pH at commonly recommended therapeutic dosages).
(5) Low doses of furosemide.

f. Drugs which alkalinize urine include:

(1) Sodium bicarbonate.
(2) Sodium lactate.
(3) Sodium acetate.
(4) Potassium citrate.
(5) Acetazolamide.
(6) Chlorothiazide.

3. ARTIFACTS

a. Contamination of urine with urease-producing bacteria from the distal urethra, genital tract or environment may result in alkalinization of urine.

b. Loss of CO_2 from samples stored at room temperature tends to alkalinize urine samples.

c. Detergents and disinfecting agents in collection containers may alkalinize urine.

d. Administration of therapeutic doses of furosemide tends to acidify urine.

II. GLUCOSE

A. INDICATIONS
1. DIAGNOSTIC

a. Although a small quantity of glucose is normally present in urine (2 to 10 mg/100 ml in man), the quantity is insufficient to be detected by screening tests commonly used as a part of routine urinalyses.

ALGORITHM for GLUCOSURIA

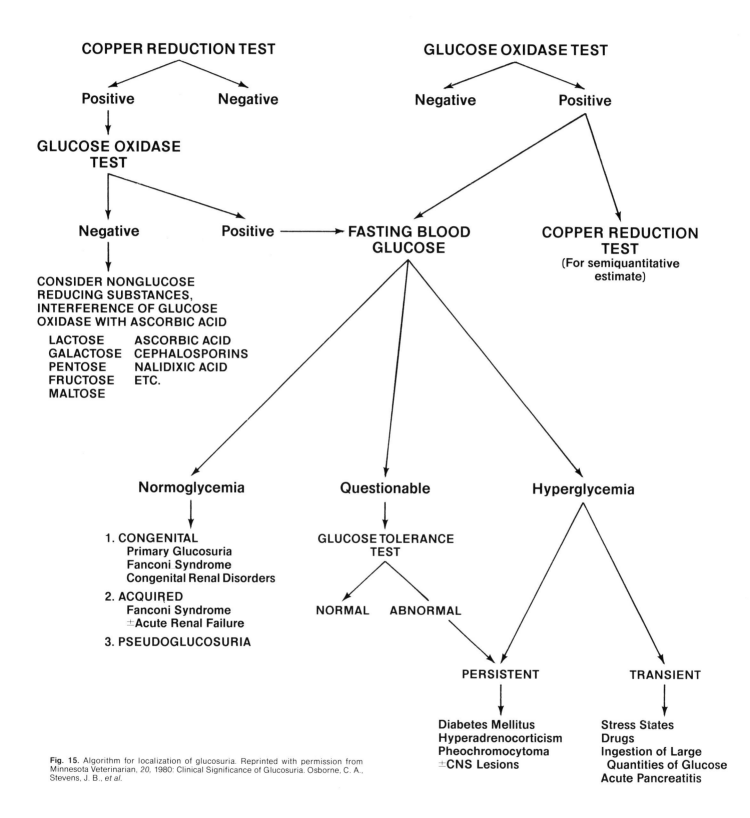

Fig. 15. Algorithm for localization of glucosuria. Reprinted with permission from Minnesota Veterinarian, *20,* 1980: Clinical Significance of Glucosuria. Osborne, C. A., Stevens, J. B., *et al.*

b. Detection of glucosuria should prompt consideration of hyperglycemic and normoglycemic states which may be physiologic or pathologic (Figure 15).

c. Test strips have been designed to detect reduction of the quantity of glucose normally present in urine as a result of consumption by bacterial pathogens. These tests have been associated with many false positive reactions in man, but have not been evaluated in dogs or cats. We have had no experience with them.

2. THERAPEUTIC

a. The dosage of insulin given to patients with diabetes mellitus is commonly influenced by semiquantitative measurements of urine glucose. Although the concentration of urine glucose is related to the concentration of blood glucose, the relationship may be influenced by many variables. Periodic evaluation of blood glucose concentration is recommended to confirm impressions based on evaluation of urine glucose concentration.

b. Detection of urine glucose is commonly used as a qualitative index of response to therapeutic osmotic diuresis induced by parenteral administration of hypertonic dextrose (so-called intensive osmotic diuresis).

B. METHODOLOGY

1. Colorimetric tests based on glucose oxidase activity.

a. Dipsticks and reagent tapes impregnated with glucose oxidase and several other reagents are available from commercial sources.

(1) Although these enzymatic tests for detection of urine glucose are technically easy to perform, they involve interrelated enzymatic reactions that occur in stepwise fashion (Figures 16-18). Reliable results are dependent on adherence to the manufacturer's recommendations for use.

(2) Although different chromogens are present in various tests, the intensity and shade of colors are reported to be roughly proportional to the quantity of glucose in urine. Color scales for comparison are provided by manufacturers.

(3) Glucose oxidase enzyme reacts specifically with glucose; the enzyme will not react with nonglucose-reducing substances (*see* discussion on Colorimetric Tests Based on Copper Reduction, page 7.7). The tests incorporate colorimetric indicators that may react, however, with nonglucose substances. Conversely, some substances may inhibit the test reaction.

(4) Glucose oxidase is a labile protein and, therefore, test strips do not have an indefinite shelf life, as indicated by an expiration date on their container.

(5) Test results may be influenced by temperature. Pilot studies performed at the University of Minnesota on canine urine with a known concentration of glucose in water (0, 100, 250, 500, 1,000, and 2,000 mg/dl) revealed that almost 25% of the samples refrigerated at 6° C and immediately tested at room temperature (21° C) with Clinistix® were falsely negative. There were no false negative results following testing samples at refrigeration temperature with TesTape® when color comparisons were made at 60 seconds. These data indicate that refrigerated samples should be warmed to room temperature before evaluation for glucose with enzyme-dependent tests requiring short

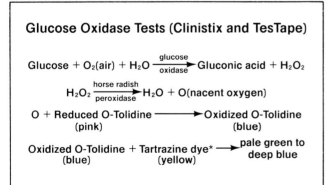

Glucose Oxidase Tests (Clinistix and TesTape)

$$Glucose + O_2(air) + H_2O \xrightarrow[oxidase]{glucose} Gluconic\ acid + H_2O_2$$

$$H_2O_2 \xrightarrow[peroxidase]{horse\ radish} H_2O + O(nacent\ oxygen)$$

O + Reduced O-Tolidine (pink) ⟶ Oxidized O-Tolidine (blue)

Oxidized O-Tolidine (blue) + Tartrazine dye* (yellow) ⟶ pale green to deep blue

Fig. 16. Interrelationship of reagents in Clinistix and TesTape and their reaction with urine glucose. *Tartrazine dye is incorporated into TesTape only. Reprinted with permission from Minnesota Veterinarian, *20*, 1980: Clinical Significance of Glucosuria. Osborne, C. A., Stevens, J. B., *et al.*

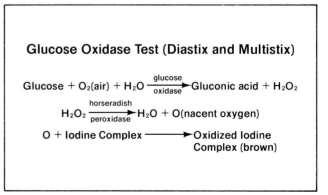

Glucose Oxidase Test (Diastix and Multistix)

$$Glucose + O_2(air) + H_2O \xrightarrow[oxidase]{glucose} Gluconic\ acid + H_2O_2$$

$$H_2O_2 \xrightarrow[peroxidase]{horseradish} H_2O + O(nacent\ oxygen)$$

O + Iodine Complex ⟶ Oxidized Iodine Complex (brown)

Fig. 17. Interrelationship of reagents in Diastix and Multistix and their reaction with urine glucose. Reprinted with permission from Minnesota Veterinarian, *20*, 1980: Clinical Significance of Glucosuria. Osborne, C. A., Stevens, J. B., *et al.*

reaction times (10 seconds). The manufacturers of Chemstrip® (read at 30 to 60 seconds) indicate that test results for glucose are not affected by temperatures between 4° and 37° C.

(6) The sensitivity of glucose oxidase tests is also influenced by pH and concentrations of inhibitors (ascorbic acid, etc.).

(7) Because many variables have the potential to affect the validity of the test, appropriate caution must be used in interpretation of semiquantitative results.

b. Clinistix® (Ames Company).

(1) Dry, solid-state reagent pads attached to a plastic strip contain glucose oxidase, peroxidase, and a colorimetric indicator (orthotoluidine). A red background dye is used to provide an easily matched negative color (see Figure 16).

(2) Color reactions are matched at 10 seconds.

(3) Three positive color blocks are light (100 mg/dl), medium (250 mg/dl), and dark (500 mg/dl+) purple (Table 12).

c. TesTape® (Eli Lilly Company).

(1) The test is based on the same principle as that used for Clinistix®; the active ingredients are the same (see Figure 16). The reagents are incorporated into a tape housed in a dispenser. A yellow background dye (F.D.C. yellow #5) is used, so that positive results give various shades of green.

(2) Color reactions are matched at 60 seconds.

(3) The color scale for comparison corresponds to approximately 0, 100, 250, 500 and 2,000 mg/dl glucose (see Table 12).

d. Diastix® and Multistix® (Ames Company).

(1) The test is based on the same principle as TesTape® and Chemstrip®, but potassium iodide is used as the chromogen (see Figure 17). A light blue background dye is also incorporated into the system.

(2) Color reactions are matched at 30 seconds.

(3) A blue color is negative, while positive results are indicated by shades of green through brown to represent 100, 250, 500, 1,000 and 2,000 mg/dl glucose (see Table 12).

(4) The manufacturer indicates that Diastix® provides more reliable semiquantitative results than Clinistix®.

e. Chemstrip®.

(1) The test principle is the same as that described for Chemstrip-G® (Figure 18).

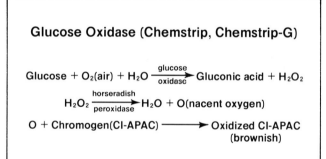

Glucose Oxidase (Chemstrip, Chemstrip-G)

$$Glucose + O_2(air) + H_2O \xrightarrow[\text{oxidase}]{\text{glucose}} Gluconic\ acid + H_2O_2$$

$$H_2O_2 \xrightarrow[\text{peroxidase}]{\text{horseradish}} H_2O + O(\text{nacent oxygen})$$

$$O + Chromogen(Cl\text{-}APAC) \longrightarrow Oxidized\ Cl\text{-}APAC \text{ (brownish)}$$

Fig. 18. Interrelationship between reagents in Chemstrips and Chemstrip-G and their reaction with urine glucose. Reprinted with permission from Minnesota Veterinarian, 20, 1980: Clinical Significance of Glucosuria. Osborne, C. A., Stevens, J. B., et al.

(2) Color reactions are kinetic; depending on the magnitude of change they are matched at one to five minutes.

(3) A gold-yellow color is normal. Positive results are indicated by changes progressing from tan to brown. The color scale on the label corresponds to 100 mg/dl(+), 250 mg/dl(++) and 1,000 mg/dl (+++) (see Table 12).

f. Chemstrip-G®.

(1) The test principle is the same as that previously described, but a different chromogen (chloro-APAC) is used to indicate positive results. This chromogen becomes a red-brown dye following oxidation with hydrogen peroxide (see Figure 18).

(2) The color reaction in Chemstrip-GK® is kinetic. The higher the glucose concentration, the longer the

Table 12

Sensitivity of Tests for Urine Glucose

TEST	Normal	<100 mg/dl	100 mg/dl	250 mg/dl	500 mg/dl	1000 mg/dl	2000 mg/dl
Chemstrip*	yellow-gold	yellow-tan (trace)	tan (+)	light brown-red(++)		dark brown (+++)	
Clinistix**	red		light purple (+)	medium purple (++)	dark purple (+++)		
TesTape***	yellow		light green (+)	darker green (++)	dark green (+++)		very dark green (++++)
Multistix**	pale blue		light green	darker green	olive	light brown	brown
Chemstrip-G*	yellow-gold	yellow-tan (trace)	tan	light brown-red	violet brown	dark brown	darker brown
Diastix**	pale blue		light green	darker green	olive	light brown	brown
Clinitest**	blue			blue green	olive green	brown	orange

*Bio-Dynamics, Indianapolis, IN 46206
**Ames Company, Elkhart, IN 46514
***Eli Lilly and Company, Indianapolis, IN 46206

reaction requires to reach an endpoint. Test results of 100 mg% or less may be read after 60 seconds, whereas values over 100 mg% are to be read after five minutes. The color is then stable and will provide accurate readings 15 minutes after the strip has been exposed to urine.

(3) A yellow color is negative. Positive results are indicated by tan (100 mg%), light brown-red (250 mg%), violet-brown (500 mg%), dark brown (1,000 mg/dl) and darker brown (2,000 mg/dl) (*see* Table 12).

2. Colorimetric tests based on copper reduction.

a. Copper reduction methods are based on color changes associated with reduction of cupric ions (blue) to cuprous oxide (orange-red) (Figure 19). Blue through green to orange is dependent on the concentration of reducing compounds (including glucose) in urine.

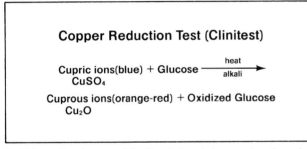

Fig. 19. Interaction of copper sulfate with reducing substances such as glucose in the presence of an appropriate environment to induce a characteristic color change. Reprinted with permission from Minnesota Veterinarian, *20*, 1980: Clinical Significance of Glucosuria. Osborne, C. A., Stevens, J. B., *et al.*

b. Clinitest® is a commercially-prepared tablet test system.

(1) Each tablet contains cupric sulfate, citric acid, sodium hydroxide and sodium carbonate.

(2) When a tablet is added to five drops of urine and 10 drops of water in a test tube, dissolution of sodium hydroxide and its interaction with citric acid provide the necessary heat for reduction of cupric ions by sugar and other reducing substances in urine.

(3) The color of the final reaction is matched to a color scale ranging from blue through green and brown to orange, corresponding to 0, 250, 500, 750, 1,000 and 2,000 mg/dl of reducing substances.

(4) Close observation is required while the reaction boils since a phenomenon termed the "pass-through" may occur with large concentrations of glucose. A concentration of more than 2,000 mg/dl causes a fleeting orange color which fades back to brown. If this color change is not observed, the

final reaction may be erroneously matched to the 1,000 mg/dl color block. Addition of two, rather than five drops of urine, may be used to avoid the "pass-through" phenomenon provided urine glucose concentration does not exceed 10 gm/dl of urine.

C. INTERPRETATION
1. SPECIFICITY OF METHODS
a. Glucose oxidase.

(1) Tests based on glucose oxidase activity are specific for glucose and will not react with nonglucose reducing substances. The tests incorporate colorimetric indicators that may react, however, with nonglucose substances.

(2) False positive reactions.

(a) Contamination of the sample or test system with small quantities of hydrogen peroxide (0.006%) will induce false positive results.

(b) Contamination of the sample or system with hydrochlorite or chlorine will give false positive results.

(c) An unidentified compound (termed pseudo-glucose) has been observed in the urine of cats with urethral obstruction.

(3) False negative reactions.

(a) Large quantities of ascorbic acid will inhibit detection of glucose by glucose oxidase tests. According to the manufacturer, Diastix® reactions are not impaired by ascorbic acid. Pilot *in vitro* studies performed in our laboratories indicated, however, that ascorbic acid is capable of interfering with this test.

(b) Outdated reagents or reagents exposed to sunlight may give erratic results.

(c) Formaldehyde (generated from methenamine) will inhibit glucose oxidase and peroxidase.

(d) Large concentrations of ketones have been reported by the manufacturer of Diastix® to depress glucose-induced color changes.

(e) Large quantities of bilirubin have been reported to inhibit Clinistix®.

(f) Addition of 300 mg of glucose to 10 ml of urine and retesting after 10 minutes may reveal some inhibitors.

(g) Reagent tapes have been reported to have an advantage over reagent pads when inhibitors are present. As urine ascends the tape by capillary action, inhibitor compounds adhere to the paper, but glucose does not. The result is development of a line of color indicative of glucosuria at the solvent front.

b. Copper reduction.

(1) Copper reduction methods are not specific for glucose.

(2) False positive reactions may be caused by a sufficient concentration of any reducing substance including:

(a) Fructose, lactose, galactose, maltose and pentoses. If necessary, thin-layer chromatography may be used to identify specifically the cause of melituria.

(b) Creatinine, homogentisic acid, and uric acid are reducing substances, but do not affect Clinitest® reactions.

(c) Ascorbic acid (endogenous and/or exogenous). Ascorbic acid is a reducing substance, and may contribute to a positive reaction.

(1) Unlike human beings, dogs and cats normally synthesize and excrete varying quantities of ascorbic acid in their urine.

(2) Ascorbic acid is sometimes used as a preservative in compounds containing drugs (such as tetracycline).

(3) Ascorbic acid is occasionally used as a urinary acidifier (although its efficacy is questionable).

(d) Conjugated glucuronates.

(1) Many compounds are conjugated with glucuronic acid in the liver prior to excretion.

(2) Conjugated bilirubin is commonly found in urine.

(3) Sufficient quantities of glucuronic acid will give a positive reaction with copper reduction tests.

(e) Certain drugs and their metabolites act as reducing substances, and, therefore, may contribute to the intensity of the color produced by copper reduction methods. Examples include:

(1) Salicylates.

(2) Large doses of penicillin.

(3) Chloral hydrate.

(f) Cephalosporin and nalidixic acid have been reported to give false positive reactions to Clinitest® in man.

(g) Formaldehyde may induce false positive reactions with Clinitest®, and therefore should not be used as a preservative for urine samples to be tested for glucose by this method.

2. SENSITIVITY OF METHODS

a. The sensitivity of all methods is influenced to varying degrees by urine specific gravity, adverse pH, interfering compounds, and suboptimum temperatures. Consult the manufacturer's product description for further information.

b. Test methods are generally more sensitive to glucose in saline than glucose in urine. The term "practical sensitivity" has been defined as being the concentration of glucose that will be detected in 90% of a fairly large number of specimens under normal conditions. Lesser quantities of glucose may be detected in most urine samples; therefore the limits of detection given as "practical sensitivity" are only intended as a general guideline.

c. Chemstrips® have been reported by the manufacturer to have a practical sensitivity of 40 mg/dl in urine samples free of ascorbic acid (i.e., human urine).

d. Clinistix® has been reported to have a practical sensitivity of less than 100 mg/dl (i.e., 90 mg/dl).

e. Multistix® has been reported to have a practical sensivity of less than 100 mg/dl (i.e., 85 mg/dl).

f. TesTape® also has been reported to have a practical sensitivity of less than 100 mg/dl (i.e., 50 mg/dl).

g. Chemstrip-G® and Diastix® (and now Multistix®) have sensitivities similar to the reagents described above, but they provide more accurate semiquantitative results. Clinistix® and TesTape® are sensitive, but provide less reliable quantitative results.

h. Clinitest® has a lower limit of sensitivity equivalent to approximately 250 mg dl. Some investigators have reported a slightly lower limit of sensitivity (150 mg/dl).

i. Ascorbic acid versus sensitivity.

(1) As previously discussed, ascorbic acid has the capacity to inhibit glucose oxidase test systems, but since it is a reducing substance it may cause or contribute to positive copper reduction tests.

(2) The amount of ascorbic acid in urine influences the degree to which it alters tests for urine glucose. The greater the concentration of glucose in urine,

the greater the quantity of ascorbic acid required to inhibit glucose oxidase tests. Likewise, the greater the concentration of ascorbic acid, the higher the reading of copper reduction test results.

(a) Ascorbic acid concentrations in urine may be estimated with a colorimetric reagent strip called C-stix® (Ames Company). It is based on color changes induced by interaction of molybdate with ascorbic acid.

(b) Ascorbic acid concentrations as low as 10-30 mg/dl will prevent detection of low concentrations of urine glucose by glucose oxidase tests.

(c) Ascorbic acid concentrations as high as 90 mg/dl have been detected in urine samples collected from dogs. We have observed an ascorbic acid concentration as high as 50 mg/dl in a cat with diabetes mellitus.

(d) These observations indicate that ascorbic acid may be present in sufficient concentration to inhibit low concentrations of urine glucose with glucose oxidase tests. Ascorbic acid may result in underestimation of the quantity of urine glucose by glucose oxidase tests and could result in insulin underdosage. Urine concentrations of ascorbic acid required to alter significantly copper reduction results in dogs and cats have not been encountered in our hospital. Ascorbic acid-induced variations in test results should be considered if urine glucose determined by glucose oxidase methods is used as an aid in titration of insulin dosage for patients with diabetes mellitus.

3. PHYSIOLOGIC GLUCOSURIA (see Figure 15)

a. Because of its molecular characteristics, glucose readily passes through glomerular capillary walls into glomerular filtrate. Almost all of the glucose in glomerular filtrate is actively reabsorbed by the proximal tubules. Only a small quantity (2-10 mg/dl, or 100-200 mg/24 hrs in man) normally appears in urine.

b. Physiologic glucosuria may occur any time the quantity of glucose in glomerular filtrate exceeds the transport capacity (so-called transport maximum or T_m) of the renal tubules for glucose. The T_m for urine glucose in dogs corresponds to a venous blood glucose concentration of approximately 170-180 mg/dl. It is obvious that hyperglycemia of a lesser magnitude may exist without glucosuria.

c. Physiologic glucosuria is usually transient in duration.

(1) Hyperglycemic glucosuria may occur following significant stress, especially in cats. This phenomenon is usually associated with the release of endogenous epinephrine and glucocorticoids, and is thought to be dependent on mobilization of glycogen stored in the liver.

(2) Hyperglycemic glucosuria has been reported in human beings following consumption of unusually large quantities of glucose. We have not observed this phenomenon in dogs or cats.

4. PHARMACOLOGIC GLUCOSURIA (see Figure 15)

a. Consult section on Glucose Interpretation, on specificity of tests (page 7.7) for additional information about false positive reactions associated with various glucose tests.

b. Hyperglycemic glucosuria may occur following parenteral administration of solutions containing sufficient quantities of glucose.

c. Varying degrees of glucosuria may be induced by parenteral administration of glucocorticoids, but in our experience this has been extremely uncommon in dogs and cats.

d. Other pharmacologic agents that have been reported to have the potential to induce glucosuria include:
(1) ACTH.
(2) Glucagon.
(3) Epinephrine.
(4) Morphine.
(5) Phenothiazines.

5. PATHOLOGIC GLUCOSURIA (see Figure 15)

a. Hyperglycemic glucosuria may be induced by several disorders including:
(1) Diabetes mellitus.
(2) Acute pancreatitis (variable).
(3) Hyperadrenocorticism (variable).
(4) CNS lesions (variable).
(5) Pheochromocytoma.

b. Normoglycemic glucosuria may be induced by several disorders including:
(1) Primary renal glucosuria.
(2) Fanconi syndrome (also called amino-diabetes).
(3) Congenital renal disorders.
(4) Acute renal failure associated with significant tubular lesions (variable).

6. INTERPRETATION OF COMBINATION TEST RESULTS (*see* Figure 15)

    a. A negative glucose oxidase test and a negative copper reduction test indicate absence of significant quantities of glucose in urine.

    b. A positive glucose oxidase test and a negative copper reduction test indicate less than 250 mg/dl of glucose in urine, or a false positive glucose oxidase reaction.

    c. A positive glucose oxidase test and a positive copper reduction test indicate glucosuria in excess of 250 mg/dl.

    d. A negative glucose oxidase test and a positive copper reduction test indicate nonglucose-reducing substances in urine.

III. KETONES

A. INDICATIONS

1. Definition: Ketones (sometimes called ketone bodies) include acetoacetic acid, acetone, and β-hydroxybutyric acid.
2. Evaluation of urine for ketones in patients with diabetes mellitus is especially important since diabetic ketonuria suggests development of diabetic ketoacidosis.
3. Evaluation of urine for ketones may aid in differentiation of a diabetic coma from therapeutically-induced insulin shock.
4. Occurrence of ketonuria in the absence of glucosuria suggests a derangement in carbohydrate metabolism characterized by excessive catabolism of lipids.

B. METHODOLOGY

1. Most tests used as a part of routine complete urinalyses for detection of ketones are based on the reaction of acetoacetic acid and acetone with nitroprusside in an alkaline environment to produce a deep purple-colored compound (*see* Figure 20).
2. Ketostix® Keto-Diastix®, Labstix®, and various Chemstrips®.

    a. These reagent strips contain test pads impregnated with sodium nitroprusside, glycine (aminoacetic acid), and an alkaline phosphate buffer (disodium hydrogen phosphate). The buffer provides an optimum pH for the reaction.

        (1) The interaction of these reagents with ketones is depicted in Figure 20.

        (2) The reactions are specific for acetoacetic acid and acetone; they will not detect β-hydroxybutyric acid. The reaction is much more sensitive to acetic acid than acetone. The following results of one study illustrate the variable sensitivity of the sodium nitroprusside reaction for different ketones in urine (Table 13).

Table 13

Sensitivity of Sodium Nitroprusside Reaction for Different Ketones in Urine

COLOR	β-HYDROXYBUTYRIC ACID	ACETOACETIC ACID	ACETONE
Neg	Neg	$\leq$ 5 mg/dl	$\leq$ 70 mg/dl
Weak	Neg	10-25 mg/dl	100-400 mg/dl
Moderate	Neg	25-50 mg/dl	400-800 mg/dl
Strong	Neg	50-150 mg/dl	800-2,000 mg/dl
Very Strong	Neg	> 150 mg/dl	> 2,000 mg/dl

    b. The color of the reagent pad should be examined at the appropriate time (15 seconds for Ames products, and 60 seconds for Bio-Dynamics products) after the immersion of the reagent strip in urine. The color of the test strips should be compared to the color scale on the label.

        (1) Positive results from beige (buff) to lavender to purple indicate ketonuria.

        (2) The intensity of color is proportional to the quantity of ketones present:

            (a) + = 5 to 40 mg/dl

            (b) ++ = 40 to 100 mg/dl

            (c) +++ = more than 100 mg/dl

Reaction of Strip and Tablet Tests for Ketonuria

Acetoacetic Acid + Sodium Nitroprusside + Glycine and Acetone

$$\xrightarrow[\text{(NaOH)}]{\text{alkaline pH}} \text{Purple colored complex}$$

Fig. 20. Reagents and biochemical events associated with positive strip and tablet tests for ketonuria.

3. Acetest® (Ames Company).

    a. Acetest® is a tablet test based on the same reactions as those described for reagent strips. In addition, lactose is added to enhance the quality of color changes.

    b. The test is performed by placing a reagent tablet on a white square piece of filter paper and placing one drop of urine on the tablet. Thirty seconds later the color of the tablet should be compared to the color scale supplied by the manufacturer. A positive reaction is indicated by a lavender to deep purple color, being dependent on the quality of the ketones present.

C. INTERPRETATION

1. SPECIFICITY

    a. The nitroprusside reaction will detect acetoacetic acid, and to a lesser degree acetone, but will not react with β-hydroxybutyric acid. Approximately 96% of the total color is due to acetoacetic acid.

    b. High concentrations of cysteine may induce a transient pink color reaction.

    c. Pyruvate has the potential to cause a blue color change but rarely is present in urine in sufficient concentration to interfere with detection of ketones.

    d. Although excretion of phenylketones in urine in concentrations equal to or greater than 100 mg/dl will cause false positive color reactions (orange-red), phenylketonuria of this magnitude is uncommon in man, and has not been reported in animals.

    e. Administration of bromosulfophthalein dye (BSP) to evaluate liver function may result in production of a color (reddish) which mimics a positive reaction for ketonuria in alkaline urine. Similar reactions with phenolsulphophthalein (PSP) would be expected.

    f. *L-DOPA* has been reported to cause false positive results in human beings (brownish-violet color).

    g. If toluene is used as a preservative, it should be used sparingly because acetone is soluble in toluene.

    h. The concentration of ketones has been reported to decrease *in vivo* as a result of urinary tract infection, and *in vitro* as a result of bacterial contamination. Bacteria may reduce the quantity of acetoacetic acid but not acetone.

2. SENSITIVITY

    a. The manufacturers indicate that the lower limit of sensitivity of these tests is approximately 5-10 mg/dl for acetoacetic acid and approximately 70 mg/dl for acetone. β-hydroxybutyric acid will not contribute to color development.

    b. It is possible to estimate crudely the quality of ketones present by using the lower limits of sensitivity and diluting the test sample until only a trace reaction can be identified. For example:

        (1) A urine sample is diluted by mixing one drop of urine with nine drops of water (1:10 dilution).

        (2) The test indicates a trace of ketones.

        (3) The actual quantity of ketones present may be calculated by multiplying the dilution factor (in this example it is 10) by the lowest limit of sensitivity (5-10 mg/dl).

        (4) 5-10 mg/dl x 10 = 50-100 mg/dl of ketones.

3. APPLIED PHYSIOLOGY

    a. During normal metabolism, fats are almost completely converted to carbon dioxide, water and energy in the liver. In the process, however, small quantities of intermediary metabolites (acetoacetic acid—also called diacetic acid, β-hydroxybutyric acid and acetone) are formed. These intermediary metabolites are metabolized by peripheral tissues of the body at a limited rate. Some are filtered by glomeruli and are almost completely reabsorbed by the renal tubules.

    b. Acetone is irreversibly formed from acetoacetic acid by nonreversible decarboxylation, whereas, β-hydroxybutyric acid is reversibly formed from acetoacetic acid.

    c. Inadequate consumption of dietary carbohydrates and/or impaired endogenous utilization of carbohydrates for energy results in a shift to increased oxidation of fatty acids. When the proportion of fatty acids metabolized for energy becomes large, utilization becomes incomplete and excessive quantities of intermediary metabolites (acetoacetic acid and its conversion products—β-hydroxybutyric acid and acetone) are formed. Catabolism of the amino acids, leucine, tyrosine and phenylalanine, may also result in increased production of acetoacetic acid. When production of these metabolites exceeds the capacity of tissues to oxidize them, they accumulate in plasma (ketosis), are filtered by glomeruli and exceed the capacity of the renal tubules to reabsorb them (ketonuria). Although ketones are excreted in urine in different relative proportions (78% β-hydroxybutyric acid, 20% acetoacetic acid and 2% acetone), detection of one indicates the presence of the others.

4. SIGNIFICANCE OF KETONURIA

a. Ketosis and ketonuria may be caused by any disorder associated with a significant shift of energy production from carbohydrates to fats.

b. Uncontrolled diabetes mellitus is the most commonly encountered form of ketonuria in dogs and cats. Urinary excretion of ketones induces systemic electro-lyte losses including hyponatremia. The loss of sodium and ketones in urine contributes to the increased osmolality of the urine due to glucose and, therefore, increases the magnitude of polyuria associated with diabetes mellitus.

c. Starvation, low carbohydrate-high fat diets (ketogenic diets), and hypoglycemic syndromes (*i.e.*, insulinomas) may also induce ketonuria.

d. Immature animals are more likely to develop ketonuria as a result of starvation than adults.

IV. BILIRUBIN

A. INDICATIONS

1. Because detection of bilirubinuria by routine urinalysis may precede clinical recognition of jaundice, bilirubi-nuria may be an early indicator of naturally-occurring disorders with the potential to induce jaundice. Lack of bilirubinuria does not exclude disorders associated with bilirubin metabolism, however.

2. Detection of abnormal quantities of bilirubin in urine may be used as a crude index of hepatotoxicity caused by potentially toxic therapeutic agents.

B. METHODOLOGY

1. Bilirubin is an unstable compound which may spon-taneously oxidize to biliverdin, especially if allowed to stand at room temperature while being exposed to light. Biliverdin will not react with commonly used tests for bilirubinuria. For this reason, urine should be evaluated within 30 minutes from the time of collection, or refrig-erated (2-8° C) in a dark environment. Urine should not be filtered or centrifuged prior to examination for bili-rubin since precipitates of calcium carbonate and calcium phosphate may absorb varying quantities of bilirubin.

2. ICTOTEST® (*see* Appendix: Ames Company)

a. Ictotest® is a tablet test based on a diazotization reaction and color change which is proportional to the quantity of bilirubin present in urine.

b. The tablets contain the following ingredients: *p*-nitro-benzole diazonium, *p*-toluene sulfonate, sulfosalicylic acid, and sodium bicarbonate. Sulfosalicylic acid pro-vides an acid environment that promotes the reaction. Addition of a small amount of sodium bicarbonate induces an effervescent mixture by reacting with sulfo-salicylic acid and producing carbon dioxide. Efferves-cence insures solution of a portion of the tablet when water is added. A bluish-violet color develops following reaction of cleaved bilirubin dypyrroles with the diazonium salt to form azobilirubin.

c. A special cellulose mat is included with the tablet whose adsorbent qualities allow bilirubin to be concen-trated at its surface.

d. To perform the test:

(1) Place five drops of urine on a square of the special test mat. Wait for each drop to be absorbed before proceeding with the next.

(2) Place a reagent tablet on the center of the moist-ened area of the mat.

(3) Allow two drops of water to flow over the tablet.

(4) Evaluate the test mat for a color change after 30 seconds.

(5) Lack of color change, pink or red colors indicate lack of bilirubin. A positive result is indicated by a blue or purple color on the mat around the tablet. The speed and intensity of color development is proportional to the degree of bilirubinuria.

(6) Color changes affecting the tablet or color changes following a lapse of 30 seconds should not be in-terpreted as positive or negative results.

(7) Avoid use of discolored tablets or tablets exposed to moisture. Exposure to moisture prior to use may induce a slow reaction between sodium bicarbonate and sulfosalicylic acid. As a result, the expected effervescent reaction created by the addition of two

drops of water during the test may be minimized or inhibited, with a reduction or inhibition of positive results.

3. ICTOSTIX® MULTISTIX® [REAGENT STICKS], etc. (*see* Appendix: Ames Company)

a. Reagent strips contain stabilized diazotized 2,4-dichloroaniline. When bilirubin is present in sufficient quantities, it reacts with this reagent to form azobilirubin and is associated with a change in color from buff to light tan or light brown. The degree of color change is dependent on the degree of bilirubinuria.

b. As mentioned, bilirubin glucuronide is much more reactive with these reagents than free bilirubin. Biliverdin cannot be detected by this method. Since bilirubin glucuronide spontaneously hydrolyzes to free bilirubin in urine samples allowed to remain at room temperature for long periods following collection, it is important to examine fresh or properly preserved specimens.

c. To perform the test:
   (1) Immerse the reagent pad of the strip into the urine sample and remove it immediately.
   (2) Tap the edge of the strip against the side of the container to remove excess urine.
   (3) After 20 seconds compare the color of the reagent pad to the color scale provided by the manufacturer.
   (4) A negative reaction is indicated by a pale lemon color (the pad is beige-colored when dry). Under favorable conditions, positive reactions are indicated by light tan (+ or 0.3 mg/dl), dark tan (++ or 0.5 mg/dl), and light brown (+++ or 1.0 mg/dl). Careful color comparisons are recommended by the manufacturer since color changes may be subtle.
   (5) Urine samples that are concentrated or discolored may be unsuitable for evaluation by this method. Questionable results should be verified by a different test method.

d. Do not use reagent tablets after the expiration date printed on label.

4. CHEMSTRIP® (6, 7 and 8) (*see* Appendix: Bio-Dynamics)

a. These reagent strips contain 2,6-dichlorobenzenediazonium-tetrafluoroborate, a buffer, and nonreactive ingredients. This test is also based on the coupling reaction of the diazonium salt with bilirubin in an acid medium to give a pink to red-violet color reaction proportional to the total bilirubin concentration.

b. To perform the test:
   (1) Immerse the reagent pad of the strip into a fresh urine sample and remove it immediately.
   (2) Tap the edge of the strip against the side of the container to remove excess urine.
   (3) After 30-60 seconds compare the color of the reagent pad to the color scale provided by the manufacturer.
   (4) A negative reaction is indicated by no color change. A change in color of the test zone from white to beige-pink indicates bilirubinuria. Varying shades of beige-pink to pale red-violet indicate slight (+ or 0.5 mg/dl), moderate (++ or 1.0 mg/dl), and heavy (+++ or 2.0 mg/dl) bilirubinuria.

5. FOAM TEST (shake test)

a. The test is based on the observation that normal, fresh urine produces white foam, while urine containing abnormal quantities of bilirubin produces yellow, yellow-green or brown foam.

b. It is not a specific phenomenon and should not be used as a substitute for a diagnostic test. Increased quantities of urobilinogen or protein may cause confusing results.

C. INTERPRETATION

1. SPECIFICITY

a. General.
   (1) The diazotization reaction is more reactive with conjugated bilirubin (more soluble) than free bilirubin (less soluble). As previously mentioned, conjugated bilirubin may spontaneously hydrolyze to free bilirubin at room temperature.
   (2) Exposure to light hastens oxidation of bilirubin to biliverdin. Biliverdin cannot be detected by the diazotization reaction.
   (3) Analysis of fresh or properly preserved samples is emphasized.
   (4) Provided selective glomerular capillary permeability to plasma proteins is not significantly altered, tests for bilirubinuria are primarily tests for conjugated bilirubin (*see* the following section on in-

terpretation of bilirubinuria for additional information).

b. Ictotest® (*see* Appendix: Ames Company).
 (1) Large quantities of ascorbic acid decrease the sensitivity of the test.
 (2) Drugs which have the capacity to change urine color may interfere with recognition of test results. For example, phenazopyridine may cause an orange to red color change.
 (3) Drugs containing phenothiazine apparently do not affect this test unless present in very large quantities.

c. Ames Company's reagent sticks (*see* Appendix).
 (1) Phenazopyridine may cause an orange to red color change.
 (2) Very large doses of phenothiazine drugs (such as chlorpromazine) have been reported to give false positive results in man.
 (3) According to the manufacturer, ascorbic acid at a concentration of 25 mg/dl or greater may cause false negative results.

d. Chemstrips® (*see* Appendix).
 (1) Large quantities of ascorbic acid in the urine may decrease the sensitivity of the test.
 (2) Drugs, such as phenazopyridine, that can color the urine red or have an intrinsic red color in acid urine may give false positive readings.
 (3) In man, it has been reported that elevated concentrations of nitrite induced by urinary tract infections result in reduced sensitivity of the test.

2. SENSITIVITY

a. Always interpret the significance of test results in light of urine specific gravity.

b. Consult the section on Glucose Interpretation for definitions of "practical" and "absolute" sensitivity.

c. Ictotest® (*see* Appendix).
 (1) The practical limit of sensitivity is 0.1 mg/dl.
 (2) Under ideal conditions the test may detect as little as 0.05 mg/dl of bilirubin in urine.

d. Ames reagent sticks (*see* Appendix).
 (1) According to the manufacturer the lower limit of sensitivity is 0.2 to 0.4 mg/dl.
 (2) Several investigators have challenged the reported

limits of sensitivity of the test.
 (3) All agree that this test is less sensitive than Ictotest.

e. Chemstrips® (*see* Appendix).
 (1) Under favorable conditions, this test may detect as little as 0.2 mg/dl of bilirubin in urine (absolute level of sensitivity).
 (2) The practical limit of sensitivity is 0.5 mg/dl.

3. APPLIED PHYSIOLOGY

a. Bilirubin is derived primarily from the catabolism of the heme component of hemoglobin in reticuloendothelial cells of the body. Small quantities are derived from pre-erythroid bone marrow sources and bone marrow metabolism.

b. Bilirubin formed as a result of degeneration of hemoglobin by reticuloendothelial cells is loosely bound to albumin and transported *via* the circulation to the liver. This form of protein-bound bilirubin is commonly called unconjugated bilirubin, free bilirubin, indirect bilirubin, slow-reacting bilirubin and hemobilirubin. Because it is bound to protein it cannot pass through glomerular capillary walls.

c. The liver removes protein-bound bilirubin from the circulation, and conjugates it with glucuronic and sulfuric acids. Conjugated bilirubin is water-soluble and passes through glomerular capillary walls. It is also called water-soluble bilirubin, direct bilirubin, bilirubin glucuronide and cholebilirubin.

d. A great majority of the conjugated bilirubin is transported to the intestinal tract in bile *via* the biliary system; however, a small amount escapes from the liver directly into the blood vascular system.
 (1) Bilirubin excreted into the small intestine is converted to urobilinogen (a colorless pigment) by intestinal bacteria. Most of the urobilinogen is ultimately oxidized to urobilin, which imparts the characteristic dark color to feces. Some of the urobilinogen, however, is reabsorbed and excreted in urine (consult the section on Urobilinogen, this chapter, page 7.30, for additional details).
 (2) Conjugated bilirubin that escapes through glomeruli may appear in urine. The renal threshold for clearance of conjugated bilirubin apparently varies from species to species, but is low in dogs. The quantity of bilirubin excreted in normal urine

is often insufficient to give a positive result, unless the urine is very concentrated.

e. At one time the origin of bilirubin normally found in urine was thought to be primarily bilirubin conjugated in the liver. Recent studies performed in dogs, however, have revealed that bilirubin may also be formed in the renal tubules following reabsorption of filtered hemoglobin. The capacity to reform tubular derived bilirubin from hemoglobin was found to be greater in males than females. Since tubular epithelial cells of dogs have been shown to contain glucuronyl transferase, the capacity of these cells to conjugate bilirubin appears probable.

f. Abnormal quantities of conjugated bilirubin in urine may be associated with:

(1) Increased production of conjugated bilirubin as a result of abnormal RBC destruction, hepatocellular disease, and/or bile duct obstruction.

(2) The combined occurrence of these disorders and renal dysfunction may lead to difficulties in quantitative interpretation of bilirubinuria because of alteration in the renal threshold for excretion of bile pigments.

g. Abnormal quantities of unconjugated bilirubin would be expected to occur in conditions associated with hyperbilirubinemia (i.e., hemolytic disease) and alteration in the selective permeability of glomerular capillaries to proteins. This hypothesis has not been substantiated in animals with experimentally-induced or spontaneously occurring diseases, however.

4. SIGNIFICANCE

a. The magnitude of bilirubinuria should always be interpreted in light of urine specific gravity.

b. Dogs.

(1) Small quantities of bilirubin are commonly observed in concentrated urine samples obtained from normal dogs.

(a) This observation is commonly attributed to a low renal threshold for bilirubin. The low renal threshold for bilirubin is associated with low plasma concentrations of bilirubin.

(b) Trace to mild reactions for bilirubin are rela-

tively common when the urine specific gravity is 1.040 or greater.

(2) Detection of bilurubin in less concentrated urine samples, or persistent bilirubinuria, should prompt consideration of disorders characterized by prehepatic, hepatic, or posthepatic disorders of bile metabolism.

(a) Bilirubinuria may precede hyperbilirubinemia.

(b) A variable degree of bilirubinuria (usually mild) may be associated with starvation and/or fever.

(c) A variable degree of bilirubinuria may be associated with intravascular hemolysis of sufficient magnitude to exceed the hemoglobin-binding capacity of haptoglobin. In this situation, bilirubinuria may be associated with renal tubular cell production of bilirubin from hemoglobin. Although damage to glomeruli may be associated with subsequent loss of unconjugated bilirubin, this mechanism is unlikely to be of clinical significance because of the magnitude of proteinuria that would be required to deliver a detectable quality of bilirubin in urine.

(d) Bilirubinuria of the greatest magnitude is usually associated with hepatocellular diseases (intrahepatic) or disorders which obstruct bile ducts (extrahepatic). A significant degree of liver disease can exist, however, in the absence of bilirubinuria.

c. Cats.

(1) Bilirubinuria in cats is uncommon.

(2) Retrospective evaluation of clinical cases admitted to the University of Minnesota Veterinary Hospital revealed that bilirubinuria was not a finding in normal cats, even when associated with highly concentrated urine samples. When discovered as a part of routine urinalysis, it should not be ignored.

(3) In the University of Minnesota series, feline bilirubinuria was associated with a variety of diseases including primary hepatic diseases, diabetes mellitus, feline infectious peritonitis, and feline leukemia-related disorders.

V. OCCULT BLOOD, HEMOGLOBIN AND MYOGLOBIN

A. INDICATIONS

1. Chemical tests for red blood cells and hemoglobin may aid in identification of the underlying cause of abnormal urine color.
2. These tests may be used to detect subvisual (occult) quantities of RBC, hemoglobin or myoglobin in urine.
3. Presence or absence of RBC, hemoglobin or myoglobin may be of value in localizing the source of proteinuria.
4. Chemical evaluation of urine for RBC may aid in interpretation of the significance of urine sediment. Since microscopic examination of urine sediment will not detect free hemoglobin released from lysed RBC, total reliance on sediment examination for semiquantitation of hematuria may result in gross underestimation of the degree of hematuria.

B. METHODOLOGY

1. OVERVIEW

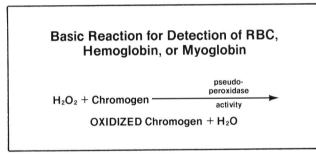

Basic Reaction for Detection of RBC, Hemoglobin, or Myoglobin

$$H_2O_2 + Chromogen \xrightarrow[\text{activity}]{\text{pseudo-peroxidase}} OXIDIZED\ Chromogen + H_2O$$

Fig. 21. Basic biochemical reaction associated with strip and tablet tests for red blood cells, hemoglobin, and myoglobin.

a. Commonly used chemical tests for rapid detection of RBC and hemoglobin are based on the pseudoperoxidase activity of the heme moiety of hemoglobin (Figure 21). Myoglobin (a heme-containing compound) also has pseudoperoxidase activity and will cause a positive test reaction. Porphyrin will not react with these tests.

b. The peroxidase activity of hemoglobin or myoglobin causes release of monomolecular oxygen from a compound containing peroxide. Transfer of monomolecular oxygen to a suitable chromogen (often o-tolidine) induces a characteristic color change. The chromogen indicator system is similar to that used in glucose oxidase-based tests for detection of urine glucose.

c. Commonly used tests are all based on this phenomenon, differing in the type of peroxide or chromogen used.

d. For screening tests, evaluation should be performed on well-mixed noncentrifuged samples.

2. HEMATEST® (*see* Appendix: Ames Company)

a. Tablet tests are essentially identical with reagent strip tests with the exception of their sensitivity. Hematest® was developed for feces, while the more sensitive reagent strips were developed for urine.

b. The source of peroxide is strontium peroxide; the chromogen is o-tolidine. A red dye is present to mask discoloration of the tablet. A mixture of tartaric acid and calcium acetate are also present to provide the most favorable pH for the reaction. Sodium bicarbonate is added so that it may react with tartaric acid to cause effervescence which aids in solubilizing the reagents and rupturing RBC. A packet of small square filter papers is supplied with the tablets.

c. In the presence of hemoglobin released from lysed RBC, free hemoglobin, or myoglobin, monomolecular oxygen is liberated from strontium peroxide and oxidizes o-tolidone to produce a blue color change.

d. To perform the test:
   (1) Place a drop of well-mixed urine on a piece of square filter paper.
   (2) Place a reagent tablet in the middle of the moistened area and then add two drops of water at a five-second interval in such a fashion as to cause the water to run over the tablet onto the filter paper.
   (3) A positive reaction is indicated by development of a distinct blue ring of color around the tablet within two minutes. The speed and intensity of the blue color change is related to the quantity of RBC, hemoglobin, and/or myoglobin in the sample. In our laboratory, the time it takes to develop the blue color is recorded as follows:

   negative = no color
   trace = slight blue color at 120 seconds
   1+ = blue color at <120 seconds
   2+ = blue color at <90 seconds

3+ = blue color at <60 seconds

4+ = blue color at <30 seconds

Color changes which develop after two minutes should be disregarded. Likewise, the color of the tablet should be ignored, even if it turns slightly blue.

3. HEMASTIX®, MULTISTIX®, etc. (see Appendix: Ames Company)

a. Like the reagent tablets just described, this reagent strip test is based on the pseudoperoxidase activity of hemoglobin or myoglobin (see Figure 21).

b. Cumen hydroperoxide is the source of peroxide; o-tolidine is the chromogen.

c. To perform the test:

(1) Dip the test strip into a well-mixed urine sample and remove it immediately.

(2) Tap the edge of the strip against the edge of the container top to remove excess urine.

(3) After 30 seconds, compare the color of the test strip to the color scale on the label.

(4) A positive reaction is indicated by a color change from colorless to blue. Based on the intensity of color change, test results may be recorded as small, moderate, or large.

4. CHEMSTRIP® (4, 5, 6, 7, and 8) (see Appendix: Bio-Dynamics Labs)

a. This reagent strip test is also based on the pseudo-peroxidase activity of RBC, hemoglobin, and myo-globin (see Figure 20).

b. Each strip contains o-tolidine (chromogen), 2,5-dimethyl-2,5-dihydroperoxyhexane (an organic source of peroxide), and a buffer.

c. Release of monomolecular (nacent) oxygen by the action of the pseudoperoxidase on the organic peroxide oxidizes o-tolidine into a green-blue dye, which in turn causes the yellow test zone to turn green.

d. Chemstrips® may permit differentiation of intact RBC from hemoglobinuria.

(1) Hemolysis of a small number of previously intact RBC on the test pad initiates production of green spots of varying numbers at that site. If large numbers of intact RBC are present, the test zone will become homogeneously green. In this situation the manufacturer suggests that the sample be diluted with physiologic saline solution to aid in differentiation of intact RBC from hemoglobinuria.

(2) A uniformly green coloration of the test pad may be caused by free hemoglobin, myoglobin or lysis of numerous RBC.

(3) Partial hemolysis of RBC may result in a diffuse green coloration of the test pad in addition to green spots produced by individual RBC. In such circumstances the test should be repeated utilizing a fresh urine sample.

C. INTERPRETATION

1. SPECIFICITY

a. False positive reactions.

(1) Peroxidase enzymes in bacteria, white cells, epithelial cells and spermatozoa are potential but very unlikely causes of false positive reactions. Studies performed using human urine indicate the high degree of improbability of these sources of peroxidase causing false positive reactions.

(2) Contamination of urine with large quantities of iodide or bromide is also a potential, but extremely unlikely, cause of false positive results.

(3) Contamination of urine samples with residues of oxidizing agents in disinfectants used to clean table tops, collection containers, etc., may cause false positive reactions.

b. False negative reactions.

(1) Failure to resuspend RBC that have settled to the bottom of the collection container may reduce or inhibit positive results.

(2) Large quantities of nitrite produced by bacteria causing urinary tract infections may delay the reaction.

(3) Use of formalin as a preservative may cause false negative results.

(4) Large quantities of endogenous or exogenous ascorbic acid (urinary acidifiers, vitamin therapy, drug preservative, etc.) may interfere with the intensity of the color reaction because it serves as an oxygen-inhibiting receptor.

c. Chemstrips® may permit differentiation between low (50 to 100/μl) to moderate ($\pm$ 300/μl) numbers of RBC from hemoglobinuria. Differentiation at higher numbers may be aided by serial dilution of the sample with physiological saline solution.

2. SENSITIVITY

a. Visual detection of blood in urine requires about 0.5 ml blood *per* liter of urine. This corresponds to approximately 2,500 RBC/μl.

b. Hematest® is reported by the manufacturers to have a practical limit of sensitivity of approximately 50 RBC/μl (50,000 RBC/ml). Other investigators have found the test to be far less sensitive than this value.

c. Hemastix® (*see* Appendix).
   (1) The absolute sensitivity for *intact RBC* is 1,000/ml (1 RBC/μl), while the practical sensitivity is 12,000 RBC/ml.
   (2) The absolute sensitivity for *free hemoglobin* is equivalent to 1,000 RBC/ml (1 RBC/μl) while the practical sensitivity is equivalent to 5,000 hemolyzed RBC/ml (5 RBC/μl).
   (3) The test is more sensitive to free hemoglobin than intact RBC.

d. Chemstrips® (*see* Appendix).
   (1) The practical limit of sensitivity for RBC is 5 RBC/μl (5,000/ml).
   (2) The practical limit of sensitivity for free hemoglobin is equivalent to 10 RBC/μl (10,000/ml).
   (3) The practical limit of sensitivity for myoglobin is 0.005 mg/dl.
   (4) The test is more sensitive to intact RBC than to free hemoglobin.

3. APPLIED PHYSIOLOGY

a. Red blood cells.
   (1) A few RBC are often present in the urine of normal dogs and cats.
   (2) Studies performed in human beings indicate that up to 5 RBC/μl (5,000/ml) are normal (so-called physiologic microhematuria). Similar quantitative determinations have apparently not been established for normal dogs, cats or other animals.
   (3) Refer to the discussion of RBC in Chapter 8, URINE SEDIMENT, for additional details.

b. Hemoglobin.
   (1) Hemoglobin is the oxygen-carrying pigment of RBC.
   (2) Normally hemoglobin released into plasma is specifically bound to a carrier protein known as haptoglobin. The molecular characteristics of haptoglobin-hemoglobin complexes are such that they normally cannot pass through glomerular capilllary walls into glomerular filtrate. Under normal conditions, plasma-derived hemoglobin does not escape into urine because the binding capacity of hemoglobin is not exceeded.
   (3) If abnormal intravascular hemolysis of sufficient magnitude to saturate the hemoglobin-binding capacity of haptoglobin occurs (variably estimated to be approximately 50-250 mg/dl of hemoglobin in dogs, and 100 mg/dl of hemoglobin in man), the tetrameric form of hemoglobin (MW = 69,000) or its smaller dimers may pass through glomerular capillary walls. At this concentration, the plasma is typically pink. If the quantity of filtered hemoglobin is in turn sufficient to exceed the reabsorptive capacity of the renal tubules, it will appear in urine.
   (4) Large quantities of free hemoglobin may also escape into urine if significant numbers of RBC undergo lysis within the excretory pathway. Hemolysis will result when the urine specific gravity is approximately 1.008 or lower, and when the urine sample is alkaline (*in vivo* or *in vitro*).

c. Myoglobin.
   (1) Myoglobin is the oxygen-carrying pigment of muscle. Although it is similar to hemoglobin, it has distinctly different physical, chemical, and immunologic properties.
   (2) Myoglobinemia of sufficient magnitude to permit detectable myoglobinuria is not normal.
   (3) Myoglobinemia and myoglobinuria may occur as a result of traumatic, toxic or ischemic injury and/or necrosis (rhabodomyolysis) to muscle cells.
   (4) Because of its molecular characteristics, myoglobin readily passes through glomerular capillary walls (MW = 17,000). Unlike hemoglobin, it is not specifically bound to a plasma carrier protein. Therefore, detectable myoglobinuria may occur when the plasma concentration of myoglobin reaches 15-20 mg/dl. This concentration is insufficient to cause a color change in plasma.

4. SIGNIFICANCE

a. Always interpret test results in association with urine specific gravity.

b. Always interpret test results in association with microscopic evaluation of urine sediment.

c. A positive chemical test for blood associated with lack of identification of RBC in urine sediment might indicate:
(1) Hemoglobinuria or myoglobinuria.
(2) Generalized hemolysis following hematuria caused by dilute and/or alkaline urine.
(3) A false positive chemical reaction.
(4) Mistaken identity of RBC in urine sediment.

d. A negative chemical test for blood-associated detection of RBC in urine sediment might indicate:
(1) Use of outdated reagents.
(2) Chemical evaluation of a poorly mixed or centrifuged urine sample.
(3) Failure of small numbers of RBC to hemolyze.
(4) Mistaken identity of RBC in urine sediment.
(5) A false negative chemical reaction.

e. Differentiation of hematuria from hemoglobinuria and myoglobinuria is of obvious importance.
(1) Centrifugation of an aliquot of a visibly discolored sample and comparison of the supernatant to an uncentrifuged aliquot of the sample may be of value.
(a) The supernatant of samples with significant hemoglobinuria or myoglobinuria will remain equally discolored.
(b) The supernatant of samples with significant hematuria will be far less discolored or normal in color.
(2) The solubility test for myoglobinuria may aid in its differentiation from hemoglobinuria.
(a) Adjust the urine pH to 7.5-8.0 with NaOH.
(b) To 5 ml of urine, add 2.8 grams of ammonium sulfate and dissolve by mixing. This will create an 80% solution.
(c) Centrifuge or filter the mixture.
(d) If the centrifugate or filtrate has an abnormal color, myoglobin is present. If only a normal color is present, the precipitated pigment is hemoglobin. If the centrifugate and precipitated pigment are abnormally colored, both are probably present.
(3) Comparison of plasma may aid in differentiation of myoglobinuria from hemoglobinuria. Patients with hemoglobinuria may have pink plasma, while the color of patients with myoglobinuria will be normal (unless both conditions are present.).
(4) Other methods which may be used to identify myoglobinuria include:
(a) Electrophoresis and immunoelectrophoresis.
(b) Spectroscopic analysis.
(c) Ultra centrifugation.
(d) Millipore filtration.

f. Hematuria.
(1) Hematuria is a nonspecific indicator of disease of the urinary tract. Once its presence has been verified, the next priority of clinical investigation is to localize its source.
(2) Refer to the discussion about hematuria in Chapter 8, URINE SEDIMENT, for additional information.

g. Hemoglobinuria.
(1) Hemoglobinuria may have a nonurinary or urinary origin.
(2) Nonurinary hemoglobinuria is associated with hemoglobinemia and may be caused by:
(a) Transfusion reactions.
(b) Immune-mediated hemolytic anemia.
(c) Babesiasis, piroplasmosis or leptospirosis.
(d) Snake venom.
(e) Hemolytic plant or chemical toxins.
(f) Drugs.
(3) Urinary hemoglobinuria is caused by extravascular hemolysis induced by dilute and/or alkaline urine.

h. Myoglobinuria.
(1) Myoglobinuria has been an uncommonly encountered disorder in dogs and cats. This may be related, at least in part, to the fact that commonly used screening tests do not permit differentiation between myoglobinuria and hemoglobinuria.
(2) Myoglobinuria may be caused by traumatic, toxic or ischemic disorders of muscles. Examples include:
(a) Crush injuries.
(b) Heat stroke.
(c) Severe or prolonged muscular exertion.
(d) Snake bites.
(e) Electric shock.
(f) Idiopathic disorders.

VI. PROTEIN

A. INDICATIONS
1. DEFINITIONS

a. Proteinuria.

Proteinuria is defined as the detection of protein in urine. Urine proteins are composed of variable quantities of plasma proteins, proteins derived from the urinary tract, and depending on the method of collection, proteins derived from the genital tract. The term "proteinuria" is usually used to imply the presence of an abnormal quantity of protein in urine. It is a laboratory finding associated with a variety of causes. The term proteinuria is preferable to albuminuria since more than forty proteins have been found in normal urine, and may also be present in disease states associated with albuminuria.

b. Bence Jones proteinuria.

Bence Jones proteinuria is defined as the presence of immunoglobulin light chains in urine.

Gamma (γ) globulins are composed of four peptide chains linked together as a unit. The inner two chains are longer and larger and are commonly called heavy chains (H chains). The outer two peptide chains are lighter and smaller and are commonly called light chains (L chains). Two types of light chains may be present, either kappa (κ) or lambda (λ). Single light chains have a molecular weight of approximately 22,000 while dimers have a molecular weight of 44,000. Because of their small size, both monomers and dimers of Bence Jones proteins readily pass through glomerular capillary walls.

Bence Jones proteins are named after Henry Bence Jones, who in 1846 emphasized the importance of their detection in urine. They are commonly associated with multiple myelomas, but may also be encountered in patients with macroglobinemia, leukemia and other disorders. It is thought that Bence Jones proteins are synthesized independently by plasma cells rather than being degradation products of abnormal myeloma proteins.

c. Orthostatic proteinuria.

Orthostatic proteinuria occurs in certain human beings during quiet, upright ambulation or standing, but not during recumbency. The excretory pattern is usually "nonselective." The cause is unknown. Orthostatic proteinuria has not been reported in animals.

d. Selective proteinuria.

Proteinuria may be characterized according to the molecular size of proteins as determined by immunoassay or Sephadex column chromatography. Mild lesions of nephrons are often characterized by the "selective loss" of albumin (MW = 69,000) and smaller globulins. With more severe damage, especially of the glomerular basement membrane, there is increased loss of higher molecular weight proteins (for example, IgG whose MW = 160,000) in addition to lower molecular weight proteins. In this instance, the proteinuria is nonselective.

2. Proteinuria may occur as a result of a variety of underlying causes as depicted by the many different types reported in the literature, including:

   a. Asymptomatic.
   b. Bence Jones.
   c. Benign.
   d. Cardiac.
   e. Exercise.
   f. False (pseudo-).
   g. Febrile.
   h. Functional (transient; intermittent).
   i. Glomerular.
   j. Inflammatory.
   k. Juvenile.
   l. Orthostatic.
   m. Paraproteinuria.
   n. Pathologic.
   o. Persistent.
   p. Physiologic.
   q. Prerenal.
   r. Renal.
   s. Tubular.
   t. Selective.

3. The quantity and composition of urine proteins vary in normal and abnormal states.

4. Evaluation of urine for protein is included as a part of complete routine urinalyses, because when interpreted in conjunction with other clinical and laboratory findings, test results often aid in detection, localization, and occasional specific identification of underlying disorders.

B. METHODOLOGY

1. OVERVIEW

a. It is more difficult to measure and identify urine proteins than serum proteins because:
   (1) Urine proteins are often present in very small quantities.
   (2) There is a large sample-to-sample variation in the amount and composition of urine protein.
   (3) Protein in urine is derived from plasma, the urinary tract and sometimes the genital tract.
   (4) Protein degradation products are concentrated by the kidney and may be measured along with intact proteins.

b. Qualitative, semiquantitative and quantitative methods are available for analysis of protein.
   (1) Most tests employed in conjunction with routine urinalyses provide qualitative and semiquantitative results.
   (2) Methods to identify and quantify urine proteins, including protein electrophoresis, gel filtration and immunochemical techniques, have been described.

2. SAMPLE COLLECTION

a. As with all tests of routine urinalysis, analyses should only be performed on samples collected prior to administration of diagnostic or therapeutic agents.

b. Although screening tests for protein may be performed on uncentrifuged samples, the test should be repeated on the supernatant of centrifuged samples to eliminate positive results caused by proteinaceous material commonly found in urine sediment (red cells, white cells, epithelial cells, casts, *etc.*).

c. Either fresh or refrigerated samples may be used. In one study, no significant change in protein concentration was detected in urine samples preserved by refrigeration at 4-10° C for four weeks.

3. SULFOSALICYLIC ACID TURBIDOMETRIC TEST

a. This test is based on the fact that sulfosalicylic acid will precipitate urine protein with resultant turbidity that is approximately equal to the quantity of protein present.
   (1) The results are semiquantitative since not all proteins form the same type of precipitate in terms of the quantity of precipitate *per* milligram of protein.
   (2) Test results may also be altered if urine turbidity is caused by nonprotein substances.
   (3) A 3-5% solution of sulfosalicylic acid mixed with an equal volume of urine is commonly used.

b. Technique:
   (1) Dissolve commercially prepared reagent tablets in water.
      (a) Bumintest® (*see* Appendix: Ames Company) contains sulfosalicylic acid and sodium sulfate (Exton's reagent).
      (b) Use four tablets/30 ml of water.
   (2) Place 10 drops of clear urine into a clean, dry test tube and add an equal amount of Bumintest® solution.
      (a) If the urine is very alkaline, add 20 drops of Bumintest® solution.
      (b) If the urine sample is cloudy:
         (1) Clear it by centrifugation or filtering.
         (2) Heat it to 38-40° C to clear it.
   (3) Thoroughly mix the solution and determine the degree of turbidity according to the following (applicable only when an equal volume of urine is mixed with an equal volume of test reagent):
      (a) No turbidity = Negative.
      (b) Faint precipitate visible against a black background = trace (5 mg/dl).
      (c) Small degree of turbidity = 1+ (10-30 mg/dl).
      (d) Moderate turbidity = 2+ (40-100 mg/dl).
      (e) Heavy turbidity = 3+ (200-500 mg/dl).
      (f) Heavy flocculation = 4+ (>500 mg/dl).
   (4) If turbidity in the original sample cannot be eliminated, compare a tube containing 10 drops of the original urine plus 10 drops of water to the tube containing the 10 drops of urine plus the 10 drops of Bumintest® solution.

4. DIPSTICK COLORIMETRIC TEST

a. These tests are based on the phenomenon called the "protein error of pH indicator dyes."
   (1) In simple terms, the test is based on the ability of amino groups of proteins to bind with and alter the color of some acid-base indicators even though their pH remains constant.
      (a) Binding of the dye is dependent on the number of free amino groups of each protein.
      (b) Albumin has more free amino groups than

globulins, hemoglobin, Bence Jones proteins, and mucoproteins. In one study it was found that the development of the same color change as that caused by a certain albumin concentration required a globulin concentration two times as high and a mucoprotein concentration three times as high.

(c) Because of reduced capacity to detect globulins, Bence Jones proteins, hemoglobin and mucoproteins, test results are semiquantitative.

(2) Tetrabromphenol blue (*see* Appendix: Ames Company) or tetrachlorophenol-tetrabromosulfonphthalein (*see* Appendix: Bio-Dynamics—Chemstrips®) is used (Figure 22).

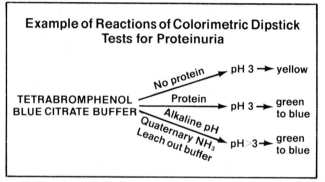

Example of Reactions of Colorimetric Dipstick Tests for Proteinuria

Fig. 22. Reagents and biochemical events associated with positive and false positive results with strip tests for proteinuria.

(a) These dyes at a pH of 3 are yellow. At a pH of 4 they are blue or green.

(b) Commercially-prepared strips are impregnated with the indicator dye and citrate buffer which maintains a pH of 3.

(c) Addition of protein in varying concentrations will result in an increasing color change from yellow to greenish-blue to blue (Ames) or yellow to light green to green (Bio-Dynamics) even though the pH remains at 3.

b. Technique.

(1) Immerse the dipstick into the urine sample and remove it immediately.

(2) Compare the color of the test strip to the color chart.

(a) Trace = approximately 5-20 mg/dl.

(b) 1+ = 30 mg/dl.

(c) 2+ = 100 mg/dl.

(d) 3+ = 300 mg/dl.

(e) 4+ ≥1,000 mg/dl.

(3) Commercial strips (*see* Appendix: Ames Company and Bio-Dynamics Laboratories) include:

(a) Albustix®—protein.

(b) Uristix®, Chemstrip® GP—protein and glucose.

(c) Combistix®, Chemstrip® 3—protein, glucose and pH.

(d) Hema Combistix®, Chemstrip® 4—protein, glucose, pH, and occult blood.

(e) Labstix®, Chemstrip® 5—protein, glucose, pH, occult blood, and ketones.

(f) Chemstrip® 6—pH, protein, glucose, ketones, bilirubin, and occult blood.

(g) Multistix®, Chemstrip® 7—protein, glucose, pH, occult blood, ketones, bilirubin, and urobilinogen.

(h) Multistix-H®, Chemstrip® 8—pH, protein, glucose, ketones, urobilinogen, bilirubin, blood, and nitrite.

c. Storage of reagent strips.

(1) Protect strips from prolonged exposure to excessive heat, humidity and light.

(2) Because the test is based on a delicate buffer system, the strips should be protected in their original container.

(3) The cap of the storage bottle should be replaced immediately following use.

5. OTHER SCREENING TESTS

a. Heller's nitric acid test, Purdy's acetic acid and heat test, and Robert's nitric acid plus magnesium sulfate test are based on denaturation and precipitation of protein.

b. These tests are not commonly used because of the potential hazard associated with the use of caustic reagents.

c. They are semiquantitative since anything insoluble in acid will give a positive result.

6. BENCE JONES PROTEINURIA

a. Electrophoretic and immunoelectrophoretic methods provide the best results.

b. The Bence Jones heat test is based on the unusual thermosolubility properties of B-J proteins.

(1) Albumin and globulins do not coagulate and precipitate out of solution until they are heated to a temperature of 56-70° C. The degree of turbidity may increase as the temperature rises.

(2) B-J proteins precipitate at 40-60° C, and redissolve as the temperature rises to 85-100° C. As the temperature cools, B-J proteins may reprecipitate at 40-60° C, and redissolve at lower temperatures. Because of this unique heat solubility, B-J proteins are sometimes called "pyroglobulins."

c. Procedure for B-J protein heat test.

(1) Place 4 ml of urine into a test tube.

(2) Add 1 ml of acetate buffer and mix.

    (a) The final pH should be 4.9 ± 0.1.

    (b) To make acetate buffer (pH 4.9, 2M), place 17.5 grams of sodium acetate trihydrate into a volumetric flask, add 4.1 ml of glacial acetic acid, and add water to 100 ml.

(3) Heat for 15 minutes in a 56° C water bath. Formation of a precipitate is indicative of B-J proteinuria.

(4) If there is turbidity or a precipitate at 56° C, heat the same tube in a boiling water bath for three minutes and check for a decrease in the amount of precipitate or turbidity. B-J proteins will redissolve at 100° C.

(5) An increase in turbidity or precipitate at boiling temperatures indicates the presence of globulins or albumin, and will mask the presence of dissolving B-J protein. In this instance, filter the contents of the tube taken directly from the boiling water bath and observe the filtrate as it cools. If it is initially clear, becomes cloudy as it cools, and then becomes clear at room temperature, the test is positive for B-J protein.

(6) A heavy precipitate of B-J protein may not redissolve on boiling. In this instance the test should be repeated with dilute urine.

(7) The urine specimen should be fresh or refrigerated since heat-coagulable protein will denature or decompose when allowed to remain at room temperature. The altered proteins may give a false positive heat test.

7. TWENTY-FOUR HOUR URINE PROTEIN DETERMINATION

a. The protein concentration in urine may vary widely from specimen to specimen. Because of unpredictable variability of protein excretion throughout the day, quantitative determinations should be based on 24-hour aliquots.

b. Samples should be collected with the aid of a metabolism cage. Preservatives such as toluene are satisfactory but the aliquot for analysis should be taken from below the toluene layered surface of the 24-hour sample.

c. Semiquantitative urine protein concentrations can be estimated with Tsuchiya's reagent using the method of Shevy and Stafford.

(1) Tsuchiya's reagent is composed of 1.5 grams of phosphotungstic acid in 95 ml of 95% ethyl alcohol. Concentrated hydrochloric acid is carefully added to make a final volume of 100 ml.

(2) A conical centrifuge tube calibrated to 0.1 ml units is required.

(3) The following step-by-step technique is recommended:

    (a) Measure the total 24-hour urine volume.

    (b) Test an aliquot of urine for protein using the Bumintest® solution as previously described.

    (c) If the protein in the urine is greater than 2+, dilute one part urine with 9 parts of distilled water.

    (d) Place 8 ml of urine (or diluted urine) into a calibrated 15 ml centrifuge tube.

    (e) Carefully stratify 5 ml of Tsuchiya's reagent over the urine.

    (f) Stopper the tube and slowly invert it three times.

    (g) Allow it to stand *exactly* one minute after inverting.

    (h) Centrifuge the mixture at 1800 RPM for 15 minutes.

    (i) Determine the volume of precipitate.

    (j) Calculate 24-hour urinary protein excretion using *0.1 cc* of precipitated protein as being equivalent to 0.036 grams of protein *per* 100 cc urine.

(4) Example:

    (a) 24-hour urine volume is 1,000 ml.

    (b) 1.8 cc of precipitated protein is formed by the test.

    (c) 18 x 0.036 grams = 0.648 grams protein excreted *per* 100 ml urine.

    (d) 0.648 grams x 10 (volume) = 6.48 grams protein excreted *per* 24 hours.

(e) If the urine was diluted, multiply the final answer by the dilution factor.

d. Biuret reagent is used in chemical laboratories to determine the quantity of protein in serum, but is too insensitive to measure smaller quantities of protein in urine unless samples are concentrated.

e. The Coomassie brilliant blue method for measurement of protein in biologic fluids has been recommended. It is a precise and sensitive method requiring spectrophotometric analysis.

C. INTERPRETATION

1. OVERVIEW

a. The interpretation of proteinuria is dependent on:
   (1) Knowledge of types and quantities of proteins normally present in urine.
   (2) Conceptual understanding of methods used to detect urine proteins.
   (3) The etiology and pathophysiology of disorders associated with proteinuria.

b. Collect urine samples for detection of urine protein prior to the administration of diagnostic and therapeutic agents.

c. Because proteinuria may be transient and of little clinical significance, verify its existence and persistence before pursuing potentially costly and time-consuming diagnostic plans to determine its cause and before initiating therapy to control or correct it.

d. Always interpret qualitative and semiquantitative tests in light of urine specific gravity.
   (1) Most screening tests for proteinuria are performed on a small volume of urine without regard to the rate of formation of urine or total volume.
   (2) For example, mild proteinuria (1+) in the presence of a low specific gravity (i.e., 1.005) implies a greater loss of protein than mild proteinuria (1+) in a more concentrated sample (i.e., SG = 1.040).

e. Before considering the underlying cause of significant proteinuria, try to localize its source.
   (1) Localization is aided by knowledge of the method of urine collection.
   (2) Localization is aided by knowledge of the composition of urine sediment (Table 14).

f. Because of significant discrepancies among various laboratory tests for proteinuria, its clinical significance should always be interpreted in association with other clinical and laboratory findings.

g. The absence of proteinuria does not eliminate the presence of renal disease or renal failure. Likewise, the severity of proteinuria is not a reliable index of the severity or reversibility of the underlying disorder.

2. SPECIFICITY OF TESTS

a. Sulfosalicylic acid turbidometric test.
   (1) Sulfosalicylic acid will precipitate urine protein with resultant turbidity that is approximately equal to the quantity of protein present.
   (2) False positive test results may be obtained if urine turbidity is caused by nonprotein substances. Positive test results may be overestimated if the degree of urine turbidity is augmented by nonprotein substances.
   (3) Radiopaque contrast agents that are excreted in urine will give a false postive reaction; radiopaque contrast agents will also increase urine specific gravity.
   (4) Massive doses of penicillin, cephalothin, cephaloridine and sulfisoxazole (Gantrisin®) have been reported to give a false positive reaction for protein with sulfosalicylic acid in man.
   (5) Highly buffered alkaline urine may give false negative reactions.
   (6) Because measurement of the degree of turbidity (i.e., 1+ to 4+) is not standardized, variability in

Table 14

Examples of Different Causes of Proteinuria

Factors	Normal Concentrated Sample	Contaminated With Hypaque*	Glomerular Disease	Urinary Tract Infection	Hemorrhage
Color	Yellow	Yellow	Yellow	Yellow	Reddish
Turbidity	Clear	Sl. cloudy	Clear	Cloudy	Cloudy
Specific gravity	1.058	1.068	1.024	1.020	1.030
pH	6.5	6.0	7.0	7.5	7.0
Glucose	Negative	Negative	Negative	Negative	Negative
Acetone	Negative	Negative	Negative	Negative	Negative
Bilirubin	Trace	Negative	Negative	Negative	Negative
Protein	1+	3+	4+	2+	2+
Occult Blood	Negative	Negative	Negative	3+	4+
RBC/HPF	1-3	0-1	Negative	100+	TNTC
WBC/HPF	0-2	None	1-3	TNTC	10-15
Casts/LPF	None	None	Occasional hyaline	None	None
Epithelial Cells	Occasional	Occasional	Occasional	Many	Moderate
Bacteria	None	None	None	Many rods	None
Crystals	None	None	None	Phosphate	Occasional phosphate

*Sulfosalicylic acid; HPF = high power field; LPF = low power field; TNTC = too numerous to count.

test results between individuals and different laboratories may occur.

(7) The preservative thymol has been reported to give a false positive protein reaction with this test.

(8) Unlike colorimetric tests, sulfosalicylic acid will detect Bence Jones proteins in urine.

b. Dipstick colorimetric test.

(1) Results are not affected by urine turbidity.

(2) The urine pH of all domestic animals is 4.5 or higher. Changes of pH within psysiologic ranges usually do not affect test results. Highly alkaline urine samples may induce false positive results if the citrate buffer system is overcome and a shift in pH occurs. This problem may be corrected by reducing the pH of extremely alkaline samples to 7 with an appropriate aliquot of acid reagent (HCl).

(3) False positive results could occur if the strip was allowed to remain in the urine sample for a sufficient period of time for the citrate buffer to be leached out.

(4) As described in the preceding discussion, colorimetric reagents are more sensitive to albumin than globulins. They may not detect Bence Jones proteins unless they are present in large quantities. Negative results are usually significant with the notable exception of pure Bence Jones proteinuria.

(5) False negative results may occur if a sample is acidified following collection.

(6) Benzalkonium (see Appendix: Zephiran®, Winthrop), a cationic quaternary ammonium surface acting antimicrobial agent, and chlorhexidine have been reported to give false positive results if sufficient residues remain in collection containers.

(7) Phenazopyridine has been reported to cause false positive reactions with Chemstrips®.

(8) Infusion of polyvinyl pyrrolidone as a plasma expander has been reported to cause false positive reactions with Chemstrips® in man.

3. SENSITIVITY OF TESTS

a. Sulfosalicylic acid turbidometric test.

(1) The range of sensitivity varies between trace (5 mg/dl) and 5,000 mg/dl+.

(2) Consult the section on Technique (page 7.21) for additional information.

b. Dipstick colorimetric tests.

(1) The range of sensitivity varies between trace (approximately 5-20 mg/dl) and 1,000 mg/dl+. Consult the section on Technique (page 7.22) for additional information.

(2) Trace positive results are commonly encountered in concentrated urine samples obtained from normal dogs and cats.

c. Four-plus reactions detected by colorimetric dipstick and turbidometric tests may be as little as 0.5 to 1.0 grams/100 ml; however, it is not possible to estimate the quantity of protein present beyond this quantity.

(1) We have evaluated dogs with generalized glomerular disease characterized by 4+ dipstick and sulfosalicylic test reactions that have excreted as little as 1 gram and as much as 35 grams of protein in their urine per 24 hours.

(2) Quantitation of 4+ screening test reactions for urine protein requires determination of the quantity of protein excreted in urine per 24 hours.

4. APPLIED PHYSIOLOGY

a. Renal handling of protein.

(1) Although the precise mechanisms by which proteins are handled by the kidneys are still not completely understood, the major variables involved are:

(a) Glomerular selective permeability.

(b) Tubular reabsorption and disposal of absorbed proteins.

(2) Glomerular permeability.

(a) The glomerulus functions as a sieve, which increasingly restricts the passage of macromolecules with increasing size and molecular weight. Since cells, most proteins, and lipoproteins are too large to pass through glomerular capillary walls, they are retained within the vascular compartment and are not present in glomerular filtrate in significant quantities. Most substances in glomerular filtrate have a molecular weight of less than 68,000 (see Table 3). Thus glomerular filtrate is qualitatively, but not quantitatively, similar to plasma with respect to the concentration of electrolytes and small molecular weight substances.

(b) Although the ability of substances to traverse glomerular capillary walls is related to their molecular weight and size, it is becoming increasingly evident that renal hemodynamics, electrical charge, and perhaps their shape also influence the degree to which they are filtered.

(3) Tubular reabsorption and disposal of absorbed proteins.

  (a) Normally only a small quantity of protein is present in glomerular filtrate. In one study in dogs, the quantity of protein in proximal tubular fluid was 10-15 mg/dl or less.

  (b) Filtered proteins are absorbed and subsequently degraded by tubular epithelial cells.

    (1) On the basis of clinical and experimental studies in man and animals, it has been hypothesized that a small amount of albumin is filtered by glomeruli. Greater than 90% of the filtered albumin is absorbed by the cells of the proximal tubule and digested therein. Polypeptides and amino acids generated by hydrolysis of albumin by lysosomal cathepsins are in part retained by the cells, and in part returned to the circulation. Trace amounts of albumin are excreted in normal urine.

    (2) Current evidence indicates that absorption of protein from glomerular filtrate occurs almost exclusively in the proximal tubules. Because the absorptive-digestive capacity of proximal tubular epithelial cells is limited, large quantities of filtered protein resulting from glomerular disease saturate this mechanism and cause proteinuria.

    (3) The renal tubules degrade a variety of hormones including parathormone, insulin, growth hormone, and thyrotropic hormone.

b. Proteins originating from the urinary tract.

  (1) It has been estimated that 40-60% of the proteins normally present in urine originate from the distal tubules and collecting ducts (Tamm-Horsfall mucoprotein), the epithelial lining of the lower urinary tract and the genital tract.

  (2) The urothelium may also secrete immunoglobulins, especially IgA, as a part of local host defenses against ascending urinary tract infection.

5. NORMAL VERSUS ABNORMAL

a. Normal urine contains very small quantities of protein.

(1) In man, 40-150 mg of protein may be normally excreted into the urine *per* 24 hours. At any time, the average normal concentration of urine protein is approximately 2-8 mg/dl.

  (a) About one-third of the protein normally excreted in urine is albumin. This albumin appears to be identical to serum albumin.

  (b) The majority of proteins found in urine of normal human beings are globulins. These globulins consist primarily of alpha-1 and alpha-2 globulins, with smaller quantities of beta and gamma globulins.

(2) Relatively little data are available concerning the normal quantity of protein in the urine of animals.

  (a) In one study of healthy Beagle dogs, less than 500 mg of protein was detected in urine *per* 24 hours.

  (b) In another study, the range of protein concentration in urine obtained from normal dogs was 0-560 mg/l.

  (c) In a study of normal male and female Beagle dogs:

    (1) The mean 24-hour protein loss was 70 mg (range = 24-197 mg) using the Coomassie brilliant blue method of protein determination.

    (2) The mean 24-hour protein loss was 38 mg (range = 8-151 mg) using the trichloroacetic acid-Ponceau method.

    (3) The mean protein concentration in random samples was approximately 24 mg/dl (range = 4-95 mg/dl). ·

    (4) Significant difference in urine protein concentration was not found among samples collected by midstream voluntary voiding, cystocentesis, or catheterization.

    (5) Protein concentrations in urine from male and female dogs were not significantly different when collected by catheterization or cystocentesis.

    (6) A significantly greater protein concentration was found in urine voluntarily voided from male dogs (28 mg/dl±21) than female dogs (19 mg/dl±13).

  (d) Wide ranges in normal values probably occur as a result of biologic variability and differences in methods used for the detection and quantification of protein.

(3) The protein content of most normal urine samples is below the sensitivity of commonly used tests for proteinuria.

    (a) Therefore persistent proteinuria of sufficient quantity to be detected by usual laboratory tests should be investigated (Figure 23).

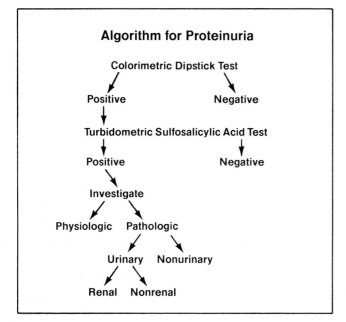

Algorithm for Proteinuria

Fig. 23. Algorithm for verification and localization of proteinuria.

    (b) Trace and 1+ results are commonly observed with colorimetric dipstick tests used in concentrated urine samples obtained from normal dogs and cats. If reagent strip tests are used as screening tests for proteinuria, positive findings should be confirmed with a test based on different biochemical reactions, such as the sulfosalicylic acid test (*see* Figure 23).

b. Abnormal.

(1) Proteinuria usually refers to an abnormally increased amount of protein in urine, and is often an important sign of urinary and/or extraurinary disease.

(2) Proteins excreted in disease states are generally related to serum proteins.

    (a) Albumin constitutes approximately 60-90% of protein excreted in urine in most disease states.

    (b) Smaller-sized globulins (alpha-1) are usually present in greater concentration than larger globulins.

    (3) Although the origin of protein cannot be consistently predicted on the basis of the quantity of protein detected by urinalysis, persistent proteinuria in moderate to large quantities which occurs in the absence of hematuria or pyuria indicates the presence of generalized glomerular disease. Likewise, detection of proteinuria in association with pyuria and hematuria indicates hemorrhage or inflammation. Hemorrhage or inflammation may be associated with infection, but is not pathognomonic for it. The combination of proteinuria, pyuria, and hematuria should prompt urine culture to assess further the likelihood of infection.

6. LOCALIZATION OF CAUSES OF PROTEINURIA

a. The clinical significance of proteinuria is sometimes difficult to assess because it may occur in association with a variety of urinary and extraurinary disorders (*see* Table 14).

b. Once persistent proteinuria has been verified, the following scheme of localization is suggested (*see* Figure 23):

(1) Physiologic (functional) proteinuria.

(2) Pathologic proteinuria.

    (a) Nonurinary proteinuria.

    (b) Urinary proteinuria.

        (1) Renal proteinuria.

        (2) Nonrenal proteinuria.

7. PHYSIOLOGIC (FUNCTIONAL) PROTEINURIA

a. Physiologic or functional proteinuria is usually transient in duration, disappearing as soon as the underlying cause is eliminated. It is sometimes called benign proteinuria.

b. Physiologic proteinuria may occur in association with strenuous and unaccustomed exercise including convulsions and racing.

(1) Exercise proteinuria is usually associated with concomitant hematuria, sometimes casts, and occasionally pyuria.

(2) In man, the proteinuria induced by strenuous exercise may persist for up to three days following cessation of exercise.

(3) The magnitude of proteinuria is usually mild, and

is caused by increased excretion of albumin and some globulins.

  (4) The etiopathogenesis of exercise proteinuria is unknown.

   (a) The fact that it is not associated with decreased tubular reabsorption of amino acids, ribonuclease, and glucose suggests that it is associated with increased glomerular permeability rather than decreased tubular reabsorption of proteins.

   (b) It has been hypothesized that exercise proteinuria is associated with increased acidity of blood and/or renal ischemia.

 c. Other disorders which may be associated with mild functional proteinuria include:

  (1) Emotional stress (man).

  (2) Extreme heat or cold (variable).

  (3) Fever (variable).

  (4) Production of urine during the first few days of life (man).

 d. The exact cause(s) of most forms of functional proteinuria is unknown.

8. PATHOLOGIC PROTEINURIA

 a. Nonurinary (extraurinary) proteinuria.

  (1) Nonurinary causes of proteinuria include disease processes which secondarily affect glomeruli and/or tubules.

  (2) Chronic passive congestion of the kidneys *may* induce a varying degree of proteinuria, presumably as a result of increased venous hydrostatic pressure and alteration of the selective permeability of glomerular capillary walls secondary to hypoxia. Proteinuria is not a consistent finding in these disorders. Examples include:

   (a) Congestive heart failure.

   (b) Increased intra-abdominal pressure caused by neoplasms, *etc.*

  (3) Nonurinary proteinuria may be associated with:

   (a) Excretion of hemoglobin as a result of intravascular hemolysis of sufficient magnitude to exceed the binding capacity of haptoglobin and tubular reabsorptive capacity.

   (b) Excretion of myoglobin as a result of generalized disease of muscles.

   (c) Excretion of Bence Jones proteins produced by neoplastic plasma cells.

  (4) Overload (threshold) proteinuria.

   (a) Proteinuria may be experimentally induced in dogs by injecting them with large quantities of plasma proteins. In general, this phenomenon has occurred when the plasma protein concentration was greater than 10 grams/100 ml.

   (b) A similar situation might be expected to occur in patients with hyperproteinemia caused by multiple myelomas.

  (5) Nonurinary proteinuria may occur as a result of contamination of urine with inflammatory exudate or hemorrhage originating in the genital tract.

 b. Urinary proteinuria.

  (1) Urinary proteinuria may be renal or nonrenal in origin.

  (2) Renal causes of proteinuria include:

   (a) Leakage of plasma protein through damaged glomeruli at a rate which surpasses tubular capacity to reabsorb protein.

    (1) Most forms of glomerulonephropathy are associated with a variable degree of increased permeability of the glomerular basement membrane (GBM) to protein molecules.

    (2) Since the quantity of various proteins excreted correlates inversely with their molecular weight, albumin (MW = 68,000) is the principal protein found in urine.

    (3) Minimal glomerular damage may be associated with loss of lower molecular weight proteins (albumin, β and some γ globulins). This is called "selective" proteinuria.

    (4) More severe damage may be associated with loss of higher molecular weight proteins in addition to lower molecular weight proteins. This is called "nonselective" proteinuria.

    (5) Persistent proteinuria, in moderate to large quantities, that occurs in the absence of significant hematuria and pyuria, indicates the presence of generalized glomerular disease (amyloidosis, immune-complex glomerulonephropathy, *etc.*)

    (6) Glomerulonephropathy associated with exudation of inflammatory cells may result in a combination of proteinuria, hematuria and pyuria that is difficult to distinguish from other inflammatory diseases of the urinary tract. However, this is not common.

Hypoproteinemia, hypoalbuminemia, and hypercholesterolemia provide strong support for the conclusion that persistent proteinuria is of glomerular origin.

(7) Hyaline, granular or waxy casts may be observed in urine sediment, but are not a constant finding.

(8) Unless associated with significant reduction in glomerular capillary perfusion, renal clearance of substances normally present in glomerular filtrate (urea, creatinine, phosphorus, *etc.*) will not be significantly impaired.

(b) Tubular disease may result in proteinuria as a result of impaired reabsorption and catabolism of low molecular weight proteins normally filtered by glomeruli.

(1) In pure tubular disease, the quantity of protein filtered by glomeruli is not increased.

(2) Proteins found in the urine of human beings with tubular disease include β-microglobulins, a_2-microglobulin, ribonuclease, lysozyme, insulin and light chains of immunoglobulins.

(3) Proteinuria is not a consistent finding in patients with tubular disease.

(4) Even when present, the quantity of protein excreted is small (low grade) when compared to the potential for loss of protein caused by glomerular diseases.

(c) Contamination of urine with inflammatory exudate or hemorrhage originating from the kidneys.

(d) Any combination of the aforementioned.

(3) Nonrenal causes of urinary proteinuria.

(a) Urinary proteinuria of nonrenal origin is usually associated with hemorrhagic or inflammatory lesions of the ureters, urinary bladder, and/or urethra.

(b) Contamination of urine with inflammatory exudate or blood, regardless of cause, may be associated with mild to moderate proteinuria.

(1) With regard to inflammation, the inflammatory process is associated with a significant loss of protein from dilated vessels, and degradation of large protein molecules at the site of the lesions.

(2) With regard to hemorrhage, rupture of vessels liberates protein-containing plasma, as well as red cells.

(3) The normal plasma concentration of proteins is 6-8 grams/100 ml (60-80 mg/ml). Colorimetric dipstick and sulfosalicylic acid laboratory tests for proteinuria can detect as little as 10-20 mg/100 ml.

(c) It is essential to evaluate the urine sediment when localizing the source of proteinuria (*see* Table 14). If proteinuria is detected without knowledge of the presence of hematuria or pyuria, it may be erroneously assumed that the protein originated from lesions in glomeruli and/or renal tubules.

9. PSEUDOPROTEINURIA (FALSE POSITIVE PROTEINURIA)

a. False positive reactions for protein detected by colorimetric dipsticks include:

(1) Highly alkaline buffered urine as might result after administration of alkalinizing drugs, or following degradation of urea to ammonia by urease-producing bacteria.

(2) Loss of citrate buffer from the dipstick as a result of prolonged immersion in the urine sample.

(3) Contamination of the sample with quaternary ammonium compounds.

b. False positive reactions for protein detected by sulfosalicylic acid include:

(1) Excessively turbid urine prior to initiation of test.

(2) Radiopaque contrast agents excreted in urine.

(3) Excretion of large quantities of penicillin, cephaloridine, or sulfisoxazole.

(4) Contamination of the test sample with thymol, a urine preservative.

10. FALSE NEGATIVE PROTEINURIA

a. False negative reactions for protein detected by colorimetric dipsticks include:

(1) Low to moderate amounts of Bence Jones proteins.

(2) Examination of a urine sample which has been acidified following collection.

b. False negative reactions for proteins detected by sulfosalicylic acid include:

(1) Evaluation of highly buffered alkaline urine.

(2) Inability to read the results because of urine turbidity prior to testing.

VII. UROBILINOGEN

A. INDICATIONS

1. Unlike the situation in man, we have not found routine examination of urine for urobilinogen to be particularly useful. Since use of the test has regained popularity in recent years because it is commonly included as one of the tests in multiple test reagent strips (Multistix®, Chemstrip®, *etc.*), we have included a discussion of this procedure. Tests for urine urobilinogen are not included as a part of routine complete urinalyses in our clinical laboratory.

2. Evaluation of urine for urobilinogen is typically used as a screening test for:
   a. Hepatic disorders.
   b. Hemolytic disorders.
   c. Patency of the bile duct.

B. METHODOLOGY

1. Because urobilinogen is unstable, meaningful results can only be obtained by analysis of fresh urine samples.

   a. Urobilinogen may be oxidized to urobilin (a dark greenish compound) in the bladder if urine is acid, or if exposed to light following collection.

   b. Urobilin will not result with commonly used screening tests for urobilinogen.

2. UROBILISTIX® AND MULTISTIX® (*see* Appendix)

   a. This reagent strip test is based on a modification of the standard Ehrlich's aldehyde reaction. The test pad contains strongly acid-buffered para-dimethyl aminobenzaldehyde (Figure 24). Urobilinogen reacts with this reagent to form a red condensation product.

Reaction of Urobilistix and Multistix for Urobilinogen

p-dimethyl aminobenzaldehyde + urobilinogen

$\xrightarrow{\text{acid pH}}$ red compound

Fig. 24. Reagents and biochemical events associated with positive Urobilistix and Multistix tests for urobilinogen.

b. To perform the test:
   (1) Immerse the reagent pad into a fresh urine sample and rapidly remove it.
   (2) Compare the color of the test strip to the color scale after one minute. The scale comprises five color blocks (from light yellow to dark brown) corresponding to 0.1, 1, 4, 8 and 12 Ehrlich units. One Ehrlich unit is equivalent to 1 mg/dl. The test cannot be relied upon to detect the complete absence of urobilinogen.

3. CHEMSTRIPS® (7 AND 8) (*see* Appendix)

   a. The reagent test pad on the strip is impregnated with a diazonium salt (*p*-methoxybenze-benzene diazofluoroborate) and a strong acid buffer (Figure 25). Urobilinogen reacts with the diazonium salt to form a red azodye.

Reaction of Chemstrips for Urobilinogen

p-methoxybenzene diazofluoborate + urobilinogen

$\xrightarrow{\text{acid pH}}$ red azo dye

Fig. 25. Reagents and biochemical events associated with positive Chemstrip tests for urobilinogen.

b. To perform the test:
   (1) Immerse the test pad into a fresh urine sample, and rapidly remove it.
   (2) After 30-60 seconds compare the test pad to the color scale composed of five colors (from white to pink to red) corresponding to normal urobilinogen concentration in urine, and to pathologic values of 1, 4, 8, and 12 mg/dl. Intermediate values may be estimated by interpolation. Absence of coloration or colors paler than the color for 1 mg/dl indicate a normal urobilinogen concentration. The color for the normal value corresponds to a urine urobilinogen concentration of approximately 0.4 mg/dl.

C. INTERPRETATION

1. SPECIFICITY

   a. Urobilistix® and Multistix® (*see* Appendix)
      (1) Metabolites of para-aminosalicylic acid, sulfonamides (specifically sulfisoxazole), and other compounds with aromatic amines may cause false positive reactions. They usually form brown to red condensation products.
      (2) Phenazopyridine may result in production of a red color because of marked acidity of the buffer in

the reagent pad.

(3) Metabolites normally found in varying quantities in urine, including indole, skatole and indican, may cause a false positive reaction.

(4) Oxidation of urobilinogen in stale urine samples may inhibit or reduce a positive reaction.

(5) Formaldehyde at concentrations of 200 mg/dl or higher has been reported to inhibit the reaction in human beings. Sources include urine preservatives and methenamine (a urinary antiseptic).

(6) A sufficient concentration of nitrite will depress or inhibit the reaction as a result of oxidation of urobilinogen to urobilin. Urobilin will not react with these reagents to produce a characteristic color change.

b. Chemstrips® (*see* Appendix).

(1) This test is reported to have greater specificity than tests based on Ehrlich's aldehyde reaction. It is not affected by indole, skatole or indican in physiologic or pathologic concentrations.

(2) Phenazopyridine may result in production of a red color because of the marked acidity of the buffer in the reagent pad.

(3) Oxidation of bilirubin in stale urine samples may inhibit or reduce a positive reaction.

(4) High concentrations of formaldehyde will inhibit or depress positive reactions (*see* Specificity of Urobilistix®).

(5) Nitrites have less tendency to interfere with this test than those based on Ehrlich's aldehyde reaction, although they still have the potential to do so.

(6) Bilirubin occasionally produces a pale greyish-green color after one minute (possibly due to biliverdin).

2. SENSITIVITY

a. General.

(1) Renal excretion of urobilinogen is pH dependent, being augmented in alkaline and suppressed in acid urine.

   (a) Urine urobilinogen excretion may be enhanced by administration of alkalinizing agents such as sodium bicarbonate.

   (b) Urine urobilinogen excretion may be reduced by administration of urinary acidifiers.

(2) Oral administration of antimicrobial agents may reduce the population of enteric bacteria and therefore interfere with conversion of bilirubin to urobilinogen.

b. Urobilistix® and Multistix® (*see* Appendix).

(1) These tests are not capable of detecting reduced quantities or absence of urine urobilinogen.

(2) The color block equivalent to 0.1 Ehrlich unit may be caused by urea.

(3) In the absence of nitrite, a negative reaction eliminates pathologic urobilinogenuria.

(4) A positive reaction requires further investigation because of its nonspecificity.

c. Chemstrips® (*see* Appendix).

(1) These tests are not capable of detecting reduced quantities or absence of urine urobilinogen.

(2) The practical limit of sensitivity is 1.0 mg/dl; the absolute limit of sensitivity is 0.4 mg/dl.

3. APPLIED PHYSIOLOGY

a. Following excretion into the small intestine, conjugated bilirubin is reduced to several colorless chromogens called urobilinoids by anaerobic bacteria. One of these metabolites is urobilinogen.

b. Most of the urobilinogen is excreted in the feces; however, some (estimated to be 10-20%) is absorbed in the portal venous system. Most of the absorbed urobilinogen is re-excreted into the intestinal tract by the liver (estimated to be 80%). This phenomenon is sometimes referred to as the enterohepatic circulation. A small quantity gains access to the systemic circulation, however, and if not bound to carrier proteins is filtered by glomeruli.

c. In addition to glomerular filtration, urobilinogen may gain access to the urinary tract by proximal tubular secretion. Urobilinogen present in tubular lumens may be reabsorbed by pH-dependent nonionic diffusion in the distal tubules. More bilirubin is excreted in alkaline than acid urine. In one study in dogs, raising urine pH from 5 to 8 resulted in an increase in excretion of filtered bilirubin from 30 to 200%.

d. The concentration of urobilinogen in urine is dependent on:

(1) The quantity of conjugated bilirubin transported to the intestine in bile.

(2) The efficiency of bacterial conversion of bilirubin to urobilinogen.

(3) The quantity of urobilinogen absorbed from the intestine.

(4) The efficiency of the liver in removing urobilinogen following absorption.

(5) Renal function.

e. Normal dogs and cats only excrete small quantities of urobilinogen in urine each day. Diurnal variation is common.

4. SIGNIFICANCE

a. Most investigators agree that screening tests for urobilinogen in the urine of dogs and cats are unreliable.

b. Even if the unreliability of the test is ignored, the results of semiquantitation of urine urobilinogen excretion are nonspecific.

c. Results of urine urobilinogen evaluation must always be interpreted in light of other clinical, laboratory, radiographic and biopsy findings.

d. Normal urobilinogen concentration.
   (1) Identification of normal quantities of urine urobilinogen suggests at least partial patency of the bile duct and adequate function of the enterohepatic circulation of bile pigments.
   (2) Consult the section of this chapter on Specificity and Sensitivity of Screening Test Methods (pages 86 and 87).

e. Decreased urobilinogen concentration.
   (1) Commonly used screening tests cannot be relied upon to detect reduced levels of urine urobilinogen. Absence or reduced quantities of urine urobilinogen are a common finding in normal dogs.
   (2) Potential causes of reduced urine urobilinogen concentration include:

(a) Impaired intestinal absorption of urobilinogen caused by disorders such as diarrhea or malabsorption.
(b) Inhibition of the intestinal bacterial flora by oral antimicrobial agents.
(c) Reduced excretion of bile into the intestine as a result of fasting or bile duct occlusion.
(d) Reduction in urine urobilinogen as a result of physiologic or pathologic polyuria.
(e) Excretion of acid urine.

f. Lack of urine urobilinogen.
   (1) Lack of detectable urine urobilinogen is a common finding in dogs.
   (2) Lack of urine urobilinogen may be associated with complete obstruction of the bile duct.
   (3) Refer to the prior discussion on *decreased urobilinogen concentration* for further information.

g. Increased urobilinogen concentration.
   (1) Increased production of conjugated bilirubin following hemolytic crises may be associated with hyperurobilinogenuria.
   (2) Hyperurobilinogenuria may be associated with hepatic dysfunction as a result of impairment of the enterohepatic circulation of bile pigments.
   (3) Delayed movement of intestinal contents may result in increased reabsorption and increased urinary excretion of urobilinogen.
   (4) Increased urine excretion of urobilinogen may be associated with an alkaline urine pH.

VIII. NITRITE

A. INDICATIONS

1. In human beings, detection of reduction of urinary nitrate to nitrite by certain bacterial pathogens is used as a screening test for significant bacteriuria.
2. Clinical evaluation of this test in dogs and cats revealed that it will not consistently detect significant bacteriuria, and therefore is unsuitable for use in these species.
3. The nitrate reduction test is included in this discussion because it is one of the tests incorporated into Microstix® and Chemstrip® (*see* appendix).

B. METHODOLOGY

1. The nitrate reduction test is dependent on the conver-

sion of nitrate, a metabolite normally present in urine, to nitrite by certain species of bacteria.

2. In the acid environment of the reagent strip, urinary nitrite will react with *p*-arsanilic acid to form a diazonium compound.
3. The diazonium compound in turn reacts with an indicator dye in the reagent pad to form a pink color.
4. The appearance of a pink color, regardless of intensity, has been reported to indicate the presence of 100,000 or more bacteria *per* milliliter of urine.

C. INTERPRETATION

1. The nitrate reduction test is unsuitable for screening of

dogs and cats for significant bacteriuria since it is associated with an extremely high number of false negative results.

2. *In vitro* tests indicate that the test is inhibited by ascorbic acid, a metabolite normally found in urine of dogs and cats.

3. Microstix® reagent strips may be used to screen dog and cat urine for significant bacteriuria. The nitrite portion of the strips, however, should be ignored.

Chapter 8. Urine Sediment

Urine Sediment

I. INDICATIONS

The value of microscopic examination of urine sediment in the interpretation of urinalysis is comparable to microscopic examination of blood smears in the interpretation of hemograms. Meaningful interpretation of color, specific gravity, turbidity, protein, occult blood and pH test results of routine analyses is dependent on knowledge of the composition of urine sediment. For example, a moderate degree of proteinuria in the absence of significant numbers of red cells and white cells usually indicates proteinuria of glomerular origin, whereas a moderate degree of proteinuria associated with hematuria and pyuria indicates an inflammatory response somewhere along the urinary and/or genital tract. If proteinuria is detected without knowledge of hematuria and/or pyuria, it may be erroneously assumed that the protein originated from lesions in glomeruli or tubules.

Examination of urine sediment may be considered as a form of biopsy (exfoliative cytology). Like other techniques of exfoliative cytology, the morphologic characteristics of cells, casts, crystals, bacteria, *etc.*, provide useful information, but frequently do not permit establishment of a specific diagnosis. Although disease states may be established on the basis of positive findings, they cannot always be eliminated by exclusion on the basis of negative findings. Therefore, the results of examination of urine sediment must be interpreted in combination with other clinical data including the physical and chemical composition of urine.

II. METHODOLOGY

A. In order to minimize variations in sediment examination from sample to sample, it is recommended that all steps in preparation be consistently performed in a standard fashion. Even with standardization of technique, reproducible semiquantitative results are often difficult to obtain.

B. The procedure to be followed in preparation of urine sediment for microscopic examination with a brightfield microscope is outlined (Table 15).

Table 15
Procedure for Preparation of Urine Sediment

1. Collect urine specimen in appropriate container.
2. If analysis cannot be performed within 30 minutes from time of collection, refrigerate sample.
3. Thoroughly mix specimen and transfer a standard volume (we prefer 5 ml) to a conical tip centrifuge tube.
4. Centrifuge the sample for 3-5 minutes at 1000 to 3000 RPM.
5. Remove the supernatant with a rubber-topped disposable pipette or by decanting, and save it for chemical analysis. Allow a standard volume (approximately ½ ml) of supernatant to remain in the test tube.
6. Thoroughly resuspend the urine sediment in the remaining supernatant by agitation of the tube or by "finger flipping" of the tube.
7. Transfer a drop of reconstituted sediment to a microscope slide with a rubber-topped disposable pipette and place a coverslip over it.
8. Subdue the intensity of the microscope light by lowering the condenser and closing the iris diaphragm.
9. Systematically examine the entire specimen under the coverslip with the low power objective, assessing the quantity and type (casts, cells, crystals, *etc.*) of sediment.
10. Examine the sediment with the high power objective to identify the morphology of elements and to detect bacteria.
11. Record the results.

1. COLLECTION OF SPECIMEN

a. Every effort should be made to collect an uncontaminated urine sample in an appropriate container.

b. Good test results cannot be obtained from poor samples.

c. For further details consult Chapter 4 on methods of urine collection.

2. PRESERVATION OF SAMPLE

a. Because the nature of urine sediment may be altered to a variable and unpredictable degree following elimination from the body, analysis of a freshly voided sample provides the most reliable results.

b. One of the most detrimental alterations that occur when urine is allowed to remain at room temperature following collection is a variable increase in pH secondary to proliferation of urease-producing bacterial contaminants and escape of CO_2 from urine into the atmosphere.

(1) Alkaline urine promotes lysis in red cells, casts, and especially white cells, and may alter crystal

composition as well.

(2) These changes may be minimized by the addition of preservatives, such as toluene or formaldehyde, but preservatives may interfere with one or more results of other tests included as a part of routine urinalysis.

c. If urinalysis cannot be performed within 30 minutes following collection, the sample should be refrigerated to minimize changes caused by bacterial contaminants and autolysis. Refrigerated samples are suitable for examination several hours following collection.

d. Consult the section on urine preservation in Chapter 3 for additional information.

3. MIX SPECIMEN AND TRANSFER TO CENTRIFUGE TUBE

a. Failure to mix a urine specimen adequately before removing an aliquot for centrifugation may result in loss of formed elements which rapidly settle to the bottom of the container.

b. Although most authors recommend the transfer of 10-15 ml of urine to a conical tip centrifuge tube, the actual volume is not critical. More important is the use of a consistent volume of urine each time, so that the diagnostician can develop some perspective of normal and abnormal findings at that volume. We routinely use 5 ml of urine because of difficulties associated with consistently obtaining larger volumes from animals.

c. Although round tip centrifuge tubes may be used, conical tip tubes are recommended since they facilitate removal of the supernatant by decanting.

4. CENTRIFUGE SAMPLE

a. The sample should be centrifuged at a relatively low rate of speed (1000 to 3000 RPM) for approximately 5 minutes.

b. The duration of centrifugation is less important than the speed of centrifugation, although it is recommended that both be standardized.

c. If the urine is centrifuged at high speeds, the sediment may become distorted as a result of packing in the bottom of the tube. When the packed sediment is forcefully resuspended in the supernatant, the formed elements may fragment.

5. REMOVE THE SUPERNATANT

a. The supernatant should be carefully removed from the test tube by decanting or with a rubber-topped disposable pipette and saved for chemical determinations. Care should be used not to disturb the sediment.

b. Since the concentration of formed elements detected by microscopy will be significantly influenced by the volume of supernatant allowed to remain in the test tube, every effort should be made to standardize this portion of the procedure; 0.5 ml is usually sufficient and usually remains following decanting on conical tip centrifuge tubes.

6. RESUSPEND THE SEDIMENT

a. This portion of the procedure is sometimes referred to as "reconstitution" of the sediment.

b. The button of sediment in the bottom of the centrifuge tube should be thoroughly mixed with the supernatant by flipping the tube with a finger, or by gentle aspiration and discharge from a disposable pipette.

c. If the sediment is not thoroughly reconstituted, heavy elements, such as casts, may remain in the bottom of the tube and escape detection.

d. If special water-soluble stains, such as Sternheimer-Malbin stain or Sedistain® are to be used, they should be added to the sediment at this time. One drop of stain is usually mixed with one drop of sediment.

Refer to the section on stains (page 8.3) for additional information.

7. PREPARATION OF MICROSCOPIC SLIDE

a. A drop of reconstituted sediment should be transferred to a clean microscope slide with a rubber-topped pipette. The drop to be examined should be sufficiently large to include the entire area covered by the coverslip, but not so large as to float the coverslip.

b. A coverslip should then be placed over the preparation. The use of a glass coverslip is recommended because it:
(1) Promotes the formation of a uniformly thin layer of sediment.
(2) Prevents contact of the microscope objectives with the sediment.
(3) Permits examination of sediment under oil immersion when necessary.

(4) Reduces the rate of evaporation of water.

(5) Minimizes movement of sediment.

c. A short time should be allowed for heavier elements to gravitate to the surface of the microscope slide and for fat droplets to float to the undersurface of the coverslip.

8. SUBDUE THE INTENSITY OF THE MICROSCOPE LIGHT

a. The refractive index of many formed elements in unstained urine sediment is similar to the surrounding medium. Therefore, it is recommended that the intensity of the microscope be subdued to improve contrast.

b. If necessary, the intensity of the light may be increased. If excessive light is used, however, many objects may be obscured.

c. Reduced illumination may be accomplished by lowering the microscope condenser and/or closing the substage iris diaphragm.

d. Visualization of formed and nonformed elements in the sediment will also be aided by continuously varying the fine focus adjustment of the microscope while the sediment is being examined.

e. Phase contrast microscopy and polarized light microscopy may also be considered to enhance visualization of urine sediment.

9. EXAMINATION UNDER LOW POWER MAGNIFICATION

a. Initially the entire sample should be systematically scanned with the aid of the low power objective (10x) to assess the quantity of sediment present and the suitability of the preparation.

b. Good preparations are characterized by a relatively even distribution of elements without excessive overlapping.

c. If the amount of material in the sediment appears to be excessive, it may be diluted with supernatant or physiological saline solution. This will alter semiquantitative interpretation of results, however. If excessive numbers of RBC are still causing interference with evaluation of the sediment, addition of 5% acetic acid solution will cause red cell hemolysis without destroying most other elements.

d. Semiquantitation of the contents of the sediment may be obtained by counting structures in at least ten fields and averaging the number of individual elements seen *per* low power field (same concept applies to counting *per* high power field).

e. Examination under low power magnification aids in the detection of elements which may be present in only a few microscopic fields (*i.e.*, casts, crystals, bile pigments).

f. Heavier elements, especially casts, often accumulate near the edges of the coverslip if excess fluid is placed on the slide.

10. EXAMINATION UNDER HIGH POWER MAGNIFICATION

Following examination of the specimen under low power magnification, it should be examined under high power magnification (40x). With the aid of increased magnification, the morphologic characteristics of cells (WBC, RBC, epithelial cells) and casts can often be seen. The presence of bacteria, yeasts, and lipid droplets may also be detected.

11. SOURCES OF TECHNICAL ERROR

In order to obtain meaningful results, avoid the following:

a. Examination of a contaminated sample.

b. Examination of unrefrigerated stale urine.

c. Failure to mix the sample thoroughly prior to examination.

d. Allowing the sediment to dry on the microscope slide.

e. Use of too much microscope light.

f. Careless reconstitution of sediment following centrifugation.

g. Centrifugation at excessive speeds.

h. Use of dirty or scratched microscope slides and coverslips.

i. Use of low power or high power magnification only.

12. STAINS FOR URINE SEDIMENT

a. With experience it is usually possible to evaluate most details of formed elements in urine sediment in an unstained preparation with proper preparation and illumination. However, some elements may be more easily recognized following staining.

b. Several stains have been recommended.
  (1) For general use:
    (a) Sternheimer-Malbin stain and modified Sternheimer-Malbin stain.
    (b) Sedistain® (*see* Appendix: Clay Adams).
  (2) For cellular elements:
    (a) New Methylene Blue.
    (b) Wright's stain.
  (3) For special needs:
    (a) Gram's stain (for classification of bacteria).
    (b) Sudan III or IV (for lipids).
c. Consult textbooks on clinical pathology for specific recommendations concerning preparation of stains, fixation of specimens, and staining techniques.

d. If a sufficient quantity of sediment is available, it is recommended that a portion be saved for unstained examination and a portion for staining.

e. Use of stains, such as Sedistain® or Sternheimer-Malbin stain, will dilute the sediment and alter semiquantitative evaluation of results.

f. Some stains applied to air-dried films of sediment, such as Gram's or Wright's stain, may require special preparation, such as heat fixation or protein coating of slides. These procedures require several staining and washing steps and may result in loss of variable quantities of sediment from the slide.

III. INTERPRETATION

A. OVERVIEW

1. Meaningful evaluation of urine sediment is dependent on recognition of cellular elements, casts, crystals and other objects. Evaluation of urine sediment is often more difficult than evaluation of blood smears or cytologic preparations from other organs of the body, partly due to the fact that cells may originate from the vascular system, interstitial tissue, or epithelial surfaces located in different areas of the urinary and/or genital tract. In addition, urine is an unphysiologic medium for most cells. Cells present in urine are subjected to osmotic and pH changes for varying periods which may be markedly different from their normal environment. They may also be exposed to enzymes or toxic concentrations of other metabolites excreted in urine or produced by pathogenic organisms. As a result they undergo changes in size, structure and transparency.

2. To minimize degenerative changes to urine caused by exposure to elements in sediment, urine may be centrifuged as soon as possible after voiding, followed by immediate examination of the sediment. Alternatively, it may be maintained with an appropriate preservative.

3. Although with experience it is usually possible to evaluate most details of formed elements in urine sediment in an unstained preparation with proper microscopic illumination, some elements may be more easily recognized by staining with Sternheimer-Malbin, New Methylene Blue or Sedistain®. Consult the section on stains for additional information (page 8.3).

4. Because knowledge of urine specific gravity provides useful information regarding the relative concentrations of water and elements in urine sediment, urine sediment results should always be interpreted in conjunction with urine specific gravity. In addition dilute urine (SG = 1.008 or less) may cause cell lysis.

5. The significance of cells, bacteria and amorphous debris should always be interpreted with knowledge of the method of sample collection. Cells and bacteria in non-catheterized samples may originate from the urethra and/or genital tract, as well as the bladder, ureters or kidneys. Red cells in catheterized samples or samples obtained by digital compression of the bladder may occur as a result of trauma induced by the collection technique. Knowledge of collection method is an important aid in localization of abnormalities.

6. NORMAL VERSUS ABNORMAL

a. Qualitative results.
  (1) Normal urine sediment may contain:
    (a) A few red blood cells (less than 5/HPF?).
    (b) A few white blood cells (less than 5/HPF?).
    (c) Transitional, squamous and/or tubular epithelial cells.
    (d) A few hyaline casts and/or a few granular casts.
    (e) A variety of crystals.
    (f) Spermatozoa.
    (g) Fat droplets.
    (h) Artifacts and contaminants.

(2) Identification of the following in urine sediment should be regarded as abnormal and investigated.

(a) More than a few red blood cells.

(b) More than a few white cells.

(c) Hyperplastic and/or neoplastic epithelial cells.

(d) More than a few hyaline or granular casts.

(e) Cellular (red blood cell, white cell, epithelial cell) casts, fatty casts, waxy casts, hemoglobin casts, *etc.*

(f) Cystine, tyrosine and leucine crystals (consult the section on crystalluria).

(g) Parasite ova and microfilaria.

(h) Bacteria in properly collected, transported and prepared specimens.

(i) Large numbers of yeast or hyphae.

b. Quantitative results.

(1) Large numbers of variables alter the quantitative composition of urine sediment, making stringent quantitative interpretations meaningless.

(2) Quantitative sediment composition may be influenced by one or more of the following:

(a) The volume of urine formed.

(b) Lysis of cells, crystals, casts *etc.*, by changes in pH and/or the degree of dilution of the sample.

(c) The sedimentation force which is dependent on speed of centrifugation (RPM), the radius of the centrifuge arm, and the duration of centrifugation.

(d) The volume of urine in which the sediment is resuspended and the thoroughness of reconstitution of the sediment.

(e) Dilution of the reconstituted sediment by addition of stains (Sedistain®, Sternheimer-Malbin, *etc.*).

(f) The quantity of sediment transferred to the microscope slide and subsequently examined (*i.e.*, the thickness of the film of the slide preparation). The volume of urine covered by a standard 22 mm coverslip and scanned under one high dry objective field (x570) has been estimated to be 1/30,000 ml.

(g) Staining procedures which may result in loss of variable quantities of sediment during counterstaining and washing.

(h) The ability to recognize various structures and the ability to differentiate between various types of cells, casts, crystals, *etc.*

c. Conventionally the number of red cells and the number of white cells are counted in each of at least ten microscopic fields, and are reported as the average number *per* high power microscope field (HPF). Casts are conventionally reported as the average number *per* low power field (LPF). Bacteria, parasites, crystals, sperm and other elements are usually reported as occasional, frequent or many. Because of the variables just described, the number of cells, casts and other elements observed represents a crude semiquantitative value at best.

d. As with all components of routine complete urinalysis, results of examination of urine sediment should be interpreted in combination with clinical observations and other laboratory, radiographic or biopsy data.

B. RED BLOOD CELLS

1. APPEARANCE (Figures 26-28)

a. The appearance of red blood cells is variable depending on specific gravity (osmolality), pH and sometimes the presence of bacteria. In fresh urine with a specific gravity of approximately 1.010-1.020, red cells appear typically as pale yellow refractive discs of uniform round shape (Figure 26). Red cells that have been in urine for a period of time may appear colorless as a result of loss of hemoglobin in the surrounding medium. They are smaller than leukocytes, contain no internal structure and may appear as biconcave discs (Figures 27-28). In concentrated urine they may become smaller, crenated and distorted, while in dilute urine they may appear larger, swollen and globular. In very dilute or alkaline urine, red cells undergo lysis and appear as faint shadows called "ghost" cells, or may become invisible. The probability of hemolysis cannot be precisely predicted from knowledge of specific gravity or osmolality because these measurements are influenced by the concentration of urea and other nonelectrolytes that have a negligible effect on osmotic equilibrium between red cells and the surrounding medium. *In vitro* and *in vivo* studies indicate that significant osmotic-induced hemolysis usually occurs in urine samples with a specific gravity of 1.008 or less.

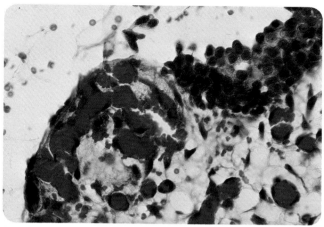

Fig. 28. Photomicrograph of a section of luminal surface of urinary bladder obtained from a dog with cystitis. Note red blood cells and transitional epithelial cells in the lumen of the bladder. Frazier-Landrum stain: high power magnification.

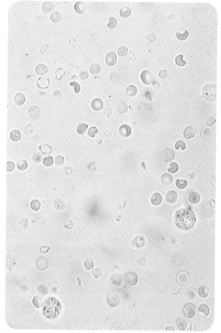

Fig. 26. Red blood cells in urine of a dog. Specific gravity was 1.029. An occasional white cell is also present. Unstained x 160 = original magnification.

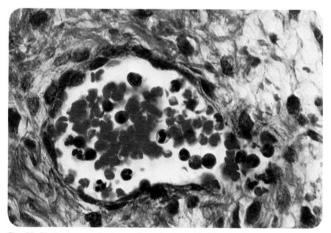

Fig. 27. Photomicrograph of a section of urinary bladder obtained from a dog with cystitis. Note escape of red blood cells and white cells from the lumen of a congested vessel. Fraizer-Landrum stain: high power magnification.

b. Because red cells have no internal structure, they sometimes resemble fat droplets, yeast cells, and amorphous urates. In contrast to RBC, however, fat droplets are variable in size and are highly refractile. Fat droplets are often out of the plane of focus of other elements in the sediment because they tend to float and often have a dark appearance when examined by subdued illumination. Yeast cells frequently contain buds, are colorless and are usually ovoid rather than round in shape. In man, amorphous urates may be red or reddish-brown in color, but are typically darker than RBC. In addition amorphous urates are variable in size and are often present in very large quantities.

2. SIGNIFICANCE

  a. Hematuria may be gross or microscopic.

  b. Gross hematuria.

    (1) If gross hematuria has been observed, determining when during the process of micturition its intensity was most severe may be helpful in localizing the source of hemorrhage.

    (2) Hematuria throughout micturition.

      (a) Patients with gross hematuria caused by renal disease usually void urine which contains blood throughout the entire period of micturition.

This occurs because the ureters enter the caudodorsal portion of the bladder and because boluses of urine are periodically discharged from the ureters into the bladder lumen.

(b) Patients with diffuse bladder lesions may also pass urine which contains blood throughout the entire period of micturition.

(c) Hematuria which occurs throughout micturition may also be observed when blood originating from severe prostatic or proximal urethral lesions refluxes from the prostatic urethra into the bladder.

(d) This pattern of hematuria could be observed in patients with a systemic clotting defect.

(e) Caution must be used to distinguish hematuria from hemoglobinuria.

(3) Hematuria at the end of micturition.

(a) Blood observed predominantly at the end of micturition suggests a focal lesion in the ventral or ventrolateral aspect of the urinary bladder.

(b) This pattern of hematuria is frequently associated with large uroliths and may be related to the fact that calculi in the dependent portion of the bladder continually traumatize this area. It may also be associated with polyps.

(c) It occurs in dogs which are sufficiently inactive to allow most of the red cells in the urine to remain in the dependent portion of the bladder lumen.

(d) Since urine contained in the uppermost portion of the bladder is forced into the urethra first, the bloody urine which has accumulated in the bottom of the bladder is voided last.

(e) This pattern of micturition could also be observed in dogs with *intermittent* gross hematuria of renal origin.

(4) Hematuria *independent* of micturition or which is most severe at the *beginning* of micturition. Hematuria which occurs independently of micturi-

tion or at the beginning of micturition usually indicates a hemorrhagic lesion in the urethra, vagina or uterus of females, or the urethra or prostate gland of males.

c. Microscopic hematuria.

(1) Hemolyzed red blood cells often cannot be detected by sediment evaluation.

(2) Results of examination of sediment for RBC should be correlated with results of chemical evaluation of urine for blood. Refer to Chapter 7 on Occult Blood for further information.

(3) An occasional RBC/HPF (< 5/HPF?) is often observed in the urine sediment of normal patients.

(4) Larger numbers of RBC in a high power microscopic field indicate hemorrhage, inflammation, necrosis, trauma or neoplasia somewhere along the urinary tract (or urogenital tract in voided samples).

d. Disorders which may be associated with hematuria include:

(1) Strenuous exercise.

(2) Iatrogenic trauma associated with palpation of the kidneys or bladder or catheterization of the bladder.

(3) Trauma.

(4) Urinary calculi in any location.

(5) Renal infarcts due to any cause (also associated with WBC, casts and protein).

(6) Infection of any portion of the urinary system (also often associated with WBC, proteinuria and bacteriuria).

(7) Benign or malignant neoplasms of any portion of the urinary system (or urogenital system in voided samples).

(8) Chronic passive congestion of the kidneys due to any cause.

(9) Diseases with systemic hemorrhagic tendencies (*i.e.*, thrombocytopenia, leptospirosis, Warfarin® toxicity, hemophilia, *etc.*).

(10) Parasites (*Dioctophyma renale, Capillaria plica,* microfilaria of *Dirofilaria immitis*).

(11) Estrus.

C. WHITE CELLS (Figures 29-32; *see* Figures 26-28)

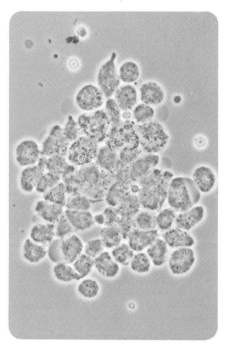

Fig. 29. Cluster of white cells. Unstained phase microscopy x 100 = original magnification.

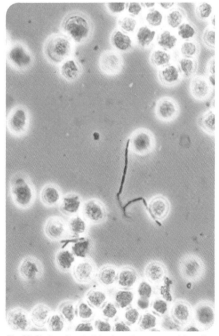

Fig. 30. Chains of bacterial rods and numerous white cells. Unstained phase contrast microscopy x 160 = original magnification.

1. APPEARANCE

a. The appearance of white cells is variable, being dependent on the type of white cells, specific gravity (osmolality), pH and the presence of toxin-producing bacteria.

(1) In fresh urine samples, WBC typically appear as spherical granular cells that are about 1½ times larger than RBC. They are usually smaller than transitional epithelial cells.

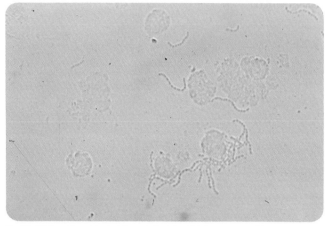

Fig. 31. White cells and bacterial cocci. Unstained high power magnification.

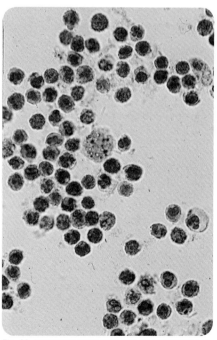

Fig. 32. Numerous white cells and an occasional epithelial cell. Sternheimer-Malbin stain x 160 = original magnification.

(2) It is sometimes possible to distinguish nuclei, but frequently their nuclei have degenerated.

(3) Granularity of white cells may be caused by disintegration of the nucleus, phagocytized material and/or granules normally present in the cytoplasm of granulocytes.

b. White cells are difficult to differentiate from renal tubular epithelial cells and a distinction between polymorphonuclear leukocytes, histocytes, lymphocytes and plasma cells is usually difficult.

c. Like RBC, white cells are rapidly lysed in alkaline or hypotonic urine.

2. SIGNIFICANCE

a. An occasional WBC/HPF ($> 5?$) may occur in normal patients.

b. Larger numbers of white cells indicate an active inflammatory lesion anywhere along the urinary tract (or urogenital tract in voided samples).

(1) The inflammatory response may be associated with varying numbers of RBC and proteinuria.

(2) Bacteria in sufficient concentration to be visualized by microscopic examination of urine, and associated with hematuria, pyuria and proteinuria indicate that the inflammatory lesion has been caused or complicated by bacterial infection. Consult the section on bacteriuria in this chapter for further information.

(3) In order to localize the site of the inflammatory process, additional information is necessary.

(4) The possibility that pyuria has occurred as a result of passage of urine through the genital tract must be considered in noncatheterized and even catheterized samples of urine. When the origin of pyuria is questionable, a urine sample obtained by cystocentesis should be re-examined.

c. Absence of pyuria usually indicates that the urinary tract is not infected. We have encountered significant asymptomatic bacteriuria without pyuria, however, in dogs and cats.

d. Pyuria (leukocyturia) is a poor index of bacteriuria and therefore is not synonymous with urinary tract infection. Although pyuria should arouse the suspicion of infection, nonseptic causes of inflammation (metabolic uroliths, neoplasms, *etc.*) should be considered.

D. EPITHELIAL CELLS (Figures 33-43; *see* Figures 28 and 32)

1. APPEARANCE

a. Renal tubular epithelial cells originate from the renal tubules. They are small, round, have a large central spherical nucleus and granular cytoplasm.

(1) Irregularity of shape and trailing cytoplasm are not pathognomonic features of renal tubular epithelial cells (Figure 39).

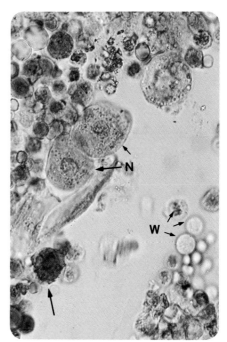

Fig. 33. Nucleated epithelial cells (N) surrounded by red blood cells, stained and unstained white cells (W), and cells of uncertain origin (arrows). Sedistain ® x 160 = original magnification.

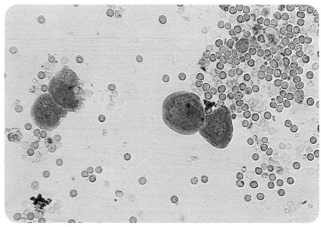

Fig. 34. Transitional epithelial cells, red blood cells, and occasional white cells. Sedistain ® x 100 = original magnification.

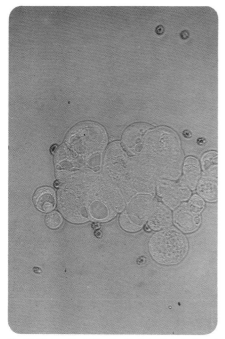

Fig. 35. Clump of transitional epithelial cells and adjacent red cells observed in the urine sediment of a dog with a transitional cell carcinoma of the urinary bladder. Unstained x 160 = original magnification.

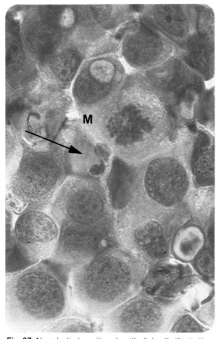

Fig. 37. Neoplastic transitional epithelial cells illustrating mitosis (M), nuclear enlargement, hyperchromasia, enlargement of nucleoli, and increased cell size. Compare to size of leukocyte (arrow). New Methylene Blue stain x 400 = original magnification.

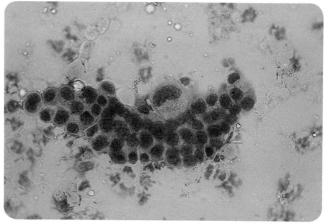

Fig. 36. Clump of transitional epithelial cells surrounded by polymorphonuclear leukocytes observed in the urine sediment of a dog with a transitional cell carcinoma of the urinary bladder. Wright's stain x 160 = original magnification.

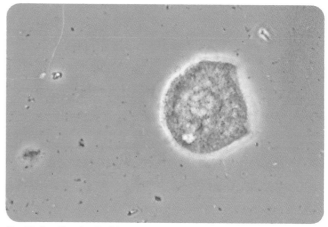

Fig. 38. Transitional epithelial cell. Unstained phase contrast microscopy x 160 = original magnification.

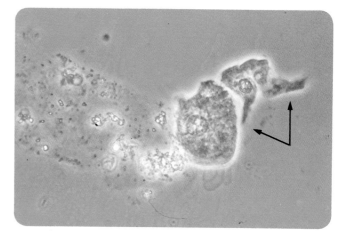

Fig. 39. Caudate epithelial cells with trailing cytoplasm (arrows). Phase contrast microscopy x 160 = original magnification.

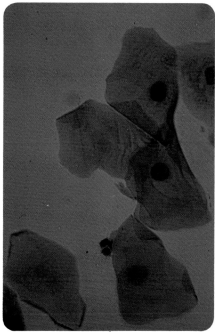

Fig. 40. Cornified squamous epithelial cells. Unstained x 400 = original magnification.

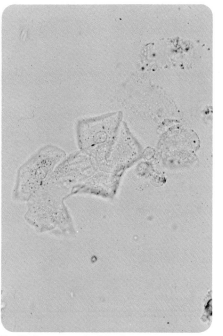

Fig. 41. Squamous epithelial cells and occasional white cell. Unstained x 160 = original magnification.

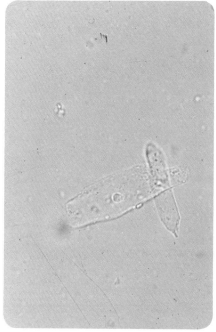

Fig. 42. Squamous epithelial cells which resemble casts. Unstained x 160 = original magnification.

(2) On occasion, cells with a brush-border (microvilli) may be observed.

(3) Contrary to often-made statements, small round cells are not a reliable index of kidney disease (unless they are contained in casts) because they cannot be readily differentiated from WBC or small transitional epithelial cells.

b. Transitional epithelial cells have a wide variation in size depending on their depth of origin in transitional epithelium. They may be pear-shaped, spindle-shaped, caudate or polygonal, and typically have granular cytoplasm (*see* Figures 32-34, and 38). They often exfoliate into urine in large numbers in association with inflammation and may be hyperplastic (*see* Figure 28).

c. Squamous epithelial cells are the largest of the cells present in normal urine sediment (*see* Figures 40-42). They are typically large, thin plate-like cells with an irregular outline and a small dense nucleus (although they may have larger vesicular nuclei). They may occur singly or in sheets.

d. Neoplastic epithelial cells may be observed in the

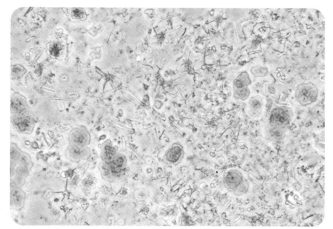

Fig. 43. Bilirubin stained cells and debris. Unstained phase microscopy x 102 = original magnification.

urine sediment of patients with transitional cell carcinomas, rhabdomyosarcomas and occasionally other types of neoplasms (*see* Figure 37). Nuclear changes indicative of malignancy are summarized in Table 16. It may be difficult to differentiate hyperplastic epithelial cells from neoplastic epithelial cells (*see* Figures 35-36).

Table 16
Abnormal Characteristics of Malignant Cells

STRUCTURAL ALTERATION OF CELLS AND THEIR NUCLEI

Nuclear Changes:
  Disproportionate enlargement of the nucleus in relation to the cytoplasm.
  Increase in chromatin content causing hyperchromasia. Structural changes
    such as aberrant chromatin patterns, elongation, irregularity in outline,
    lobulation and budding, *etc.*
  Enlargement and/or increase in number of nucleoli.
  Multinucleated cells with atypical nuclei.
  Increased mitotic activity; abnormal mitotic figures.
  Marked thickening of nuclear membrane.

Cytoplasmic Changes:
  Changes in staining reaction.
  Cytoplasmic inclusions such as pigment granules, leukocytes or
    cellular debris.
  Atypical vacuolization.

Whole Cell Changes:
  Increase in size.
  Aberrant forms.

MODIFICATION OF CELLULAR INTERRELATIONSHIPS

Irregularity of Pattern.
Anisocytosis and Anisokaryosis.
Lack of Distinct Cell Boundaries.
Dense Crowding of Cells and Nuclei.

Modifed from Prall *et al.* (1972): Cancer *29*, 1087-1089.

2. SIGNIFICANCE

a. Cuboidal epithelial cells from the renal tubules, transitional epithelial cells from the renal pelves, ureters, urinary bladder and urethra, and squamous epithelial cells from the vagina and distal urethra are commonly found in urine sediment obtained from normal dogs and cats. They are thought to occur as a result of normal attrition and exfoliation of epihelial cells.

b. Accurate data regarding the number of epithelial cells, which may normally be present in the urine of dogs and cats, are not available. Although large numbers of cells may exfoliate as a result of disease, there are more reliable methods available which should be used to confirm the presence of urinary lesions.

c. Renal tubular epithelial cells.
  (1) Originate from the renal tubules.
  (2) Are normally found in urine in relatively small numbers.
  (3) Are not a reliable index of kidney disease because they are difficult, if not impossible, to differentiate from other types of epithelial cells (unless they are incorporated into casts).

d. Transitional epithelial cells.
  (1) Originate from the renal pelvis, ureters, urinary bladder and/or urethra.
  (2) Are normally found in urine in relatively small numbers.

(3) Exfoliate into urine in large numbers as a result of inflammation or neoplasia. In these instances, they may be hyperplastic.

e. Squamous epithelial cells.
  (1) Originate from the genital tract.
  (2) Are commonly present in noncatheterized samples.
  (3) Are primarily of significance in relation to the fact that they indicate contamination of the urine sample with material from the genital tract.

f. Neoplastic epithelial cells.
  (1) May be observed in patients with transitional cell carcinomas, rhabdomyosarcomas and, less commonly, other types of neoplasms, but are not a consistent finding.
  (2) Are rarely encountered in patients with renal cell carcinomas.
  (3) Are often difficult to differentiate from non-neoplastic, hyperplastic transitional epithelial cells.

E. CASTS (Figures 44-58)

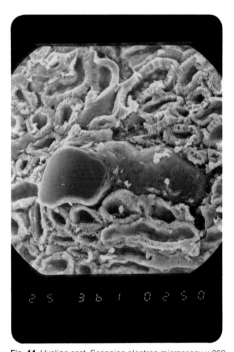

Fig. 44. Hyaline cast. Scanning electron microscopy x 360 = original magnification. Photograph courtesy of Dr. Robert F. Hammer, College of Veterinary Medicine, University of Minnesota.

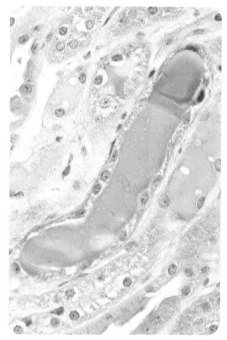

Fig. 45. Photomicrograph of a hyaline proteinaceous cast in the lumen of a renal tubule of a dog kidney. Hematoxylin and Eosin stain: high power magnification. From Stevens, J.B., and Osborne, C.A.: Urinary Casts: What is Their Significance? Minnesota Veterinarian, 18: 11-18, 1978).

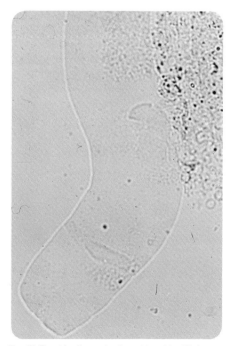

Fig. 47. Broad hyaline cast adjacent to unidentified amorphous debris. Unstained x 160 = original magnification.

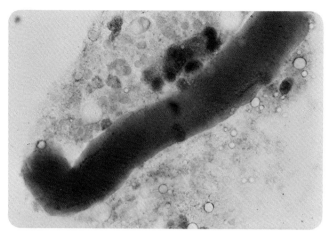

Fig. 46. Hyaline cast surrounded by cellular material, debris, and lipid droplets (unstained). New Methylene Blue stain x 160 = original magnification.

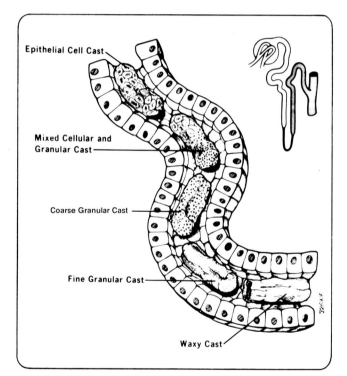

Fig. 48 Schematic illustration of transition between epithelial cell, coarse granular and waxy casts formed in the loops of Henle, distal tubules, and collecting ducts (shaded area of nephron in upper right-hand corner).

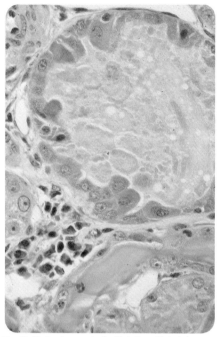

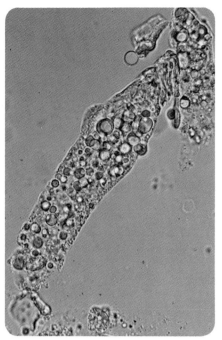

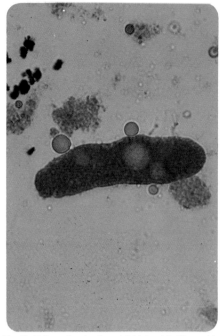

Fig. 49. Photomicrograph of a dilated renal tubule in a section of canine kidney illustrating sloughing and disintegrating of epithelial cells. These cells may become trapped into a mucoprotein matrix to form epithelial, granular or waxy casts. Hematoxylin and Eosin stain: high power magnification. From Stevens, J.B., and Osborne, C.A.: Urinary Casts: What is Their Significance? Minnesota Veterinarian, 18: 11-18, 1978).

Fig. 50. Fatty cast. Unstained x 82 = original magnification.

Fig. 51. Fatty cast and adjacent lipid droplets. The matrix of the cast is purple (New Methylene Blue stain), while lipid droplets are orange (Sudan IV stain) x 100 = original magnification.

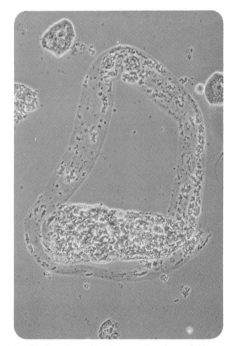

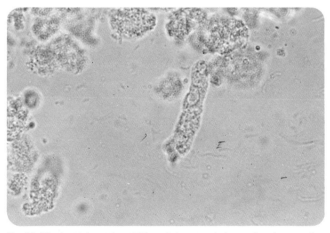

Fig. 53. Mixed granular cast containing what appears to be a cell and surrounding granular epithelial cells. Unstained x 82 = original magnification.

Fig. 52. Granular and hyaline cast. The shape of this cast suggests that it originated in the loops of Hanle and distal tubular lumen. Unstained phase microscopy x 82 = original magnification.

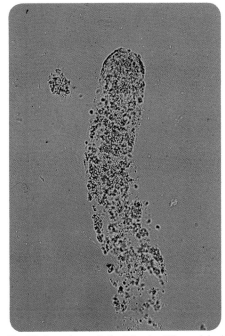

Fig. 54. Granular cast. Unstained x 160 = original magnification.

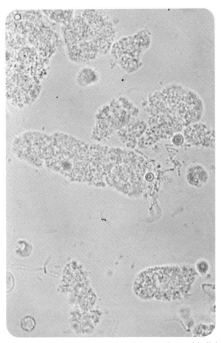

Fig. 55. Granular casts, granular disintegrating epithelial cells, bacteria and occasional white cells. Unstained x 160 = original magnification.

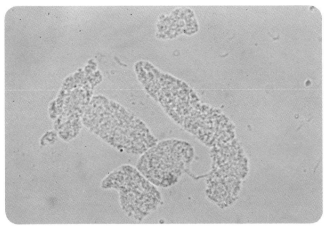

Fig. 56. Granular casts and disintegrating cells. Unstained x 160 = original magnification.

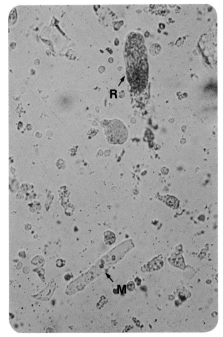

Fig. 57. Red cell casts (R) and mixed granular and waxy cast (M). Unstained x 40 = original magnification.

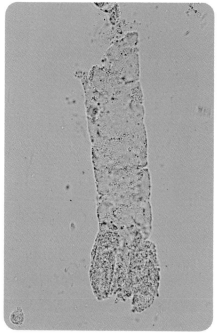

Fig. 58. Mixed granular and waxy cast. Unstained x 160 = original magnification.

1. THEORIES OF FORMATION

a. Casts are cylindrical-shaped structures composed primarily of mucoprotein (called Tamm-Horsfall mucoprotein), which by scanning electron microscopy appears as a fibrillar protein meshwork. Tamm-Horsfall mucoprotein is locally secreted by epithelial cells that line the loops of Henle, the distal tubules and the collecting ducts. Contrary to the once popular opinion, casts are not primarily composed of plasma proteins. Microdissection studies of renal tubules indicate that casts are formed in the loops of Henle, distal tubules and collecting ducts. Although the mechanism(s) responsible for the precipitation of Tamm-Horsfall mucoprotein is not understood, cast formation in these areas of nephrons is thought to be related (at least in part) to the fact that the secretion of T-H mucoprotein is limited to these sites and also that urine has the potential of reaching maximum concentration and acidity at these sites.

b. A long-time and popular theory is based on the assumption that any material or object present within the lumen of tubules at the time T-H mucoprotein gels will become incorporated into the casts. Entrapment of cells and other structures in the precipitated muco-protein matrix has been likened to entrapment of fruit and vegetables in gelatin salads.

c. It has also been hypothesized that casts may be formed by conglutination of cells and/or debris within tubular lumens.

d. Recent studies of the surface ultrastructure of casts by scanning electron microscopy indicate that erythrocytes, leukocytes and renal epithelial cells adhere to the surface of a fibrillar network of protein that subsequently surrounds the cells. The results of these structures corroborate the hypothesis that the hyaline cast is the primary structural unit of all casts.

2. APPEARANCE

a. Casts are cylindrical-shaped structures formed in tubular lumens (*see* Figures 44-45). They literally are a cast of the shape of tubular lumens.
   (1) They may have round, square, irregular or tapered ends.
   (2) The width of casts is determined by the diameter of the tubular lumens in which they are formed. Casts formed in loops of Henle or distal tubules are not as wide as those formed in collecting ducts or abnormally dilated tubules (compare Figures 46-47).

b. Accurate, precise identification of some casts by light microscopy may be difficult. To avoid misinterpretation, special stains, phase contrast microscopy and interference contrast microscopy have been advocated by various investigators.

c. Artifacts.
   (1) It has been reported that hyaline casts will dissolve in neutral urine with a specific gravity of less than 1.003.
   (2) There is an inverse relationship between the number of intact casts and urine pH. For this reason, casts are less commonly observed in alkaline urine.
   (3) High speed centrifugation and forceful reconstitution of urine may disrupt casts.

d. Casts are commonly classified on the basis of their morphologic appearance as hyaline, epithelial, granular, waxy, fatty, red blood cell, white cell, hemoglobin, broad, bile-stained and mixed casts. This classification is often of benefit in providing information about the type of lesion that is occurring in the kidneys.

e. Hyaline casts (*see* Figures 44-47, 52).

　(1) Hyaline casts are primarily composed of Tamm-Horsfall mucoprotein; they contain no inclusions.

　(2) Since the refractive index of hyaline casts is similar to the refractive index of the surrounding medium, they are usually colorless, homogeneous and semitransparent in unstained sediment.

　(3) They can be best detected in subdued light or following staining.

f. Epithelial, fatty, granular and waxy casts (*see* Figures 50-58).

　(1) A popular, but unproven, hypothesis is that epithelial, fatty, granular, and waxy casts represent different stages of degeneration of epithelial cells in casts (*see* Figure 48).

　(2) Epithelial cell casts contain varying numbers of highly refractile desquamated tubular epithelial cells which have not yet disintegrated. Scanning electron micrographs have revealed that the epithelial cells are attached to a hyaline matrix by fibrin bands. The epithelial cells characteristically have a large round central nucleus.

　(3) If lipid accumulates in the cytoplasm of cells prior to desquamation into tubular lumens, highly refractile fat droplets may be observed (*see* Figures 50-51). Such casts are sometimes called fatty casts. Verification of lipid in casts may be achieved by staining with Sudan III or IV or by examination with polarizing light microscopy (*see* Figure 51).

　(4) Once an epithelial cell cast has formed, its morphologic appearance does not remain static (*see* Figures 48, 52-54, 56-58). As a result of being deprived of oxygen and metabolites, epithelial cells degenerate. With time, cell margins become indistinct, nuclear material begins to disintegrate and coarse opaque granules appear forming a coarse granular cast. As the process of degeneration continues, fine granules are formed and the casts are called fine granular casts.

　(5) Further degeneration of the components of the epithelial cell results in the formation of a colorless, homogeneous mass with a high refractive index, sharp borders, "broken off" ends, and a dull, waxy appearance. They are called waxy casts (*see* Figures 57 and 58).

　(6) Since cellular degeneration of epithelial cells in casts occurs after cell death and desquamation, the degree (or stage) of disintegration of epithelial cells does not reflect the microscopic appearance of the tubules, but rather the duration of the disease process. Epithelial, fatty, granular and waxy casts are usually associated with diseases that cause degeneration and necrosis of tubular epithelial cells.

　(7) Granular casts may also occur as a result of degeneration of WBC in casts, and as a result of aggregation of plasma proteins in Tamm-Horsfall mucoprotein matrix.

g. Cellular casts (*see* Figure 53).

　(1) As a result of degeneration of epithelial cells or white cells, it may be impossible to distinguish cell types.

　(2) Such casts are commonly called cellular casts or cellular granular casts.

h. Red blood cell casts (*see* Figure 57).

　(1) Red blood cell casts occur in association with hemorrhage into the renal tubules.

　(2) In fresh urine they have a yellow-orange to orange-red color. This color often fades with time and the red cells may disintegrate.

　(3) Degeneration and lysis of red cells within a cast may result in a hemoglobin-induced golden-brown color and granularity.

i. Hemoglobin casts.

　(1) Hemoglobin casts may be observed following severe intravascular hemolysis and hemoglobinuria.

　(2) They are homogeneous in consistency and have a reddish color.

j. White cell casts.

　(1) White cell casts are composed of white cells and T-H mucoprotein matrix and occur when the tubules and interstitium become involved in an inflammatory process.

　(2) If the white cells degenerate before they are examined, granular casts may be formed.

k. Broad casts (*see* Figure 47).

　(1) The term broad cast refers to a wide cast formed in collecting ducts or abnormally dilated loops of Henle or distal tubules.

(2) Broad casts may be hyaline, granular or waxy in appearance.

(3) At one time broad casts were called "renal failure casts" because when present in large numbers they were often associated with renal failure.

l. Bile-stained casts represent any variety of cast that has become pigmented with bilirubin.

m. Mixed casts (*see* Figures 48, 52, 53, 57 and 58).

(1) Casts can be composed of a mixture of any of the types described.

(2) For example, casts may contain cells and granular debris (cellular granular casts) or granular debris and waxy material (granular waxy casts).

3. SIGNIFICANCE

a. Since casts are formed in the loops of Henle, distal tubules and collecting ducts, detection of significant numbers of casts in urine sediment indicates tubular involvement in an active pathologic process.

Although classification of casts according to their morphologic appearance may reflect the character of the lesion in the renal tubules, cast morphology is rarely of specific diagnostic significance.

b. Absence of casts does not rule out renal tubular disease.

c. Casts may be eliminated in urine immediately after formation or remain within tubules for varying periods undergoing varying degrees of degeneration.

d. The number of casts is not a reliable index of the severity, duration, reversibility or irreversibility of the underlying disease.

(1) For example, large or small numbers of casts may occur in patients with acute generalized renal disease because the casts tend to be discharged into the urine in intermittent showers.

(2) On the other hand, only a few casts may be observed in the urine of patients with chronic, progressive, generalized nephritis.

(3) Large numbers of casts always indicate active generalized renal disease, which is usually acute, but may be reversible or irreversible.

(4) Small numbers of casts may occur in patients with acute or chronic generalized renal disease.

e. Clinical observations have revealed that a few hyaline or granular casts (less than approximately 1 to 2/low power field in moderately concentrated urine) in the sediment of otherwise normal patients are not a reliable index of significant renal damage.

(1) Under these circumstances, a few casts are of no apparent diagnostic or prognostic significance.

(2) Although casts indicate some pathologic change in the renal tubules, this change may be minor, transitory and reversible.

f. Hyaline casts.

(1) There has been a general consensus that hyaline casts are commonly seen in association with renal and extrarenal causes of proteinuria. The proposed mechanism of hyaline cast formation in these situations is that serum proteins in urine promote aggregation of Tamm-Horsfall mucoprotein.

(2) Hyaline casts may be associated with mild or severe disease.

g. Epithelial, fatty, granular, and waxy casts.

(1) These casts may be associated with diseases (infarction, ischemia, nephrotoxins, *etc.*) that cause degeneration and necrosis of tubular epithelial cells.

(2) Contrary to earlier reports, waxy casts are not a consistent finding in patients with amyloidosis and are not composed of amyloid.

(3) Granular casts may also arise from precipitation of plasma proteins in T-H mucoprotein matrix and as a result of degeneration of WBC.

h. Red cell casts.

(1) Red blood cell casts occur in association with hemorrhage into renal tubules.

(2) Although observation of RBC in urine sediment does not indicate the site of bleeding, observation of RBC casts indicates that the kidneys are involved.

i. White cell casts.

(1) White cell casts occur in association with tubulo-interstitial inflammation.

(2) As was the situation with RBC, observation of white cells in urine sediment does not indicate the site of inflammation. Observation of white cell casts indicates renal involvement in the inflammatory process.

(3) Absence of white cell casts does not exclude inflammation of the renal tubules.

j. Broad casts.
(1) Broad casts indicate obstruction of more than one nephron if they originate in collecting ducts. At one time they were called "renal failure casts" because when present in large numbers they were often associated with renal failure.
(2) Broad casts may also originate in abnormally dilated tubules of nephrons.

k. Bilirubin casts are associated with bilirubinuria (*see* Chapter 7, section on Bilirubin, for additional information).

F. BACTERIA (Figure 59; *see* Figures 30-32, 84).

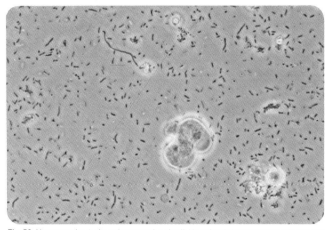

Fig. 59. Numerous bacteria and an occasional cell. Unstained phase contrast microscopy x 102 = original magnification.

1. APPEARANCE

a. Bacterial rods and cocci may be observed in urine sediment if present in sufficient numbers.

b. The sediment must be examined under high dry or oil immersion magnification.

c. Single cocci are more difficult to identify than rods and chains of cocci because they are often mistaken for Brownian movement of amorphous crystals.

d. *In vitro* studies suggest that rod-shaped bacteria must be present in quantities equal to or greater than 30,000/ml before they can be reproducibly detected in urine samples. An even greater number of cocci may be required to permit detection.

e. Because bacteria are apparently not affected by centrifugation at 1,000 to 3,000 RPM for 3-5 minutes in the same fashion as cells, crystals, casts, *etc.*, either centrifuged or uncentrifuged samples may be examined. Centrifugation and examination of urine sediment may, however, facilitate detection of bacteria in the cytoplasm of phagocytic inflammatory cells.

f. Phase contrast microscopy may facilitate detection of bacteria in unstained samples (*see* Figures 30 and 59).

g. A variety of stains (New Methylene Blue, Gram's stain, *etc.*) may facilitate detection and identification of rods and cocci in urine samples.

2. SIGNIFICANCE

a. Microscopic examination of urine for bacteria should be used to complement rather than substitute for qualitative and quantitative urine culture.

b. Bacteriuria may or may not be significant depending on the method of urine collection and the length of time between collection and examination.

c. Interpretation versus collection method.
(1) Normally urine is sterile until it reaches the mid-urethra.
(2) The urethra of dogs, and presumably cats, contains a resident population of bacteria, which are greatest in number at the distal end of the urethra. Most of these organisms are Gram positive, but Gram negative bacteria and mycoplasms are also present.
(3) The significance of bacteria identified in voided or catheterized urine samples should be interpreted with caution because samples collected by these methods may be contaminated with resident bacteria located in the distal urethra and genital tract.
(4) The concept of significant bacteriuria was introduced to allow differentiation between harmless bacterial contaminants of urine and pathogenic organisms causing infectious disease of the urinary system. The number of bacteria considered to be significant varies with the method of urine collection (and perhaps with species).
(a) This concept is based on the observation that a high bacterial count in a properly collected and prepared urine sample is indicative of urinary tract infection.
(b) In human beings, urine bacterial counts in excess of 100,000 organisms of a single species *per* milliliter are considered to be significant. The detection of 10,000 to 100,000 bacteria of a

single species *per* milliliter in catheterized or midstream urine samples is interpreted as suspicious of bacterial infection. Less than 10,000 bacteria *per* milliliter in voided or catheterized samples usually represent contaminants.

(c) Clinical studies of urine cultures performed at the University of Minnesota Veterinary Hospital utilizing the calibrated loop technique for quantitative urine culture have revealed that noncatheterized and catheterized midstream urine samples obtained from infected and noninfected dogs have similar numbers of bacteria as that reported for man.

(d) Recent studies of cats at the University of Minnesota indicate that feline urine may normally inhibit bacterial growth to a greater degree than canine or human urine. In other words, numbers of bacteria considered to be contaminants, or suspicious of urinary tract infections in dogs and man, may be indicative of urinary tract infections in cats. Further studies must be performed before meaningful generalities can be established.

(5) Since urine in the urinary bladder is normally sterile, detection of any bacteria in an appropriately stored and processed sample collected by cystocentesis is indicative of significant bacteriuria. Doubt may exist concerning the association of low numbers of bacteria and contamination from the skin, collection container, *etc.* Therefore, 100 to 1,000 organisms in samples collected by cystocentesis should be regarded as questionable.

d. Interpretation versus length of time between collection and examination.

(1) The significance of detection of bacteria in urine samples allowed to incubate at room temperature prior to examination is unknown.

(a) Pathogens and/or contaminants may continue to proliferate or be destroyed.

(b) *In vitro* bacteria growth or destruction is not synonymous with *in vivo* conditions.

(2) Detection of bacteria in improperly preserved samples warrants re-examination of a fresh specimen.

e. Microscopic examination versus bacterial numbers.

(1) Rod-shaped bacteria may be seen in unstained or stained preparations of urine when numbers are approximately 30,000 or greater. Larger numbers of cocci may be required to permit detection.

(2) The results of a study in dogs were interpreted to indicate that detection of bacteria in more than one oil immersion field was an indication of 100,000 bacteria *per* milliliter or more.

f. Significant bacteriuria is usually, but not invariably, associated with varying degrees of hematuria, pyuria and proteinuria (*i.e.*, an inflammatory response).

g. Lack of detection of bacteria in urine sediment does not exclude their presence.

G. YEASTS AND FUNGI (Figures 60-63)

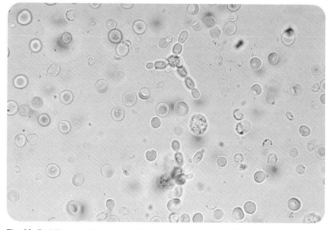

Fig. 60. Budding yeast in urine sediment of a cat, surrounded primarily by red blood cells. An occasional white cell is also present. Unstained x 160 = original magnification.

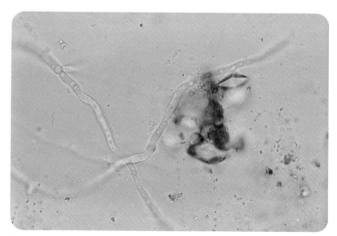

Fig. 61. Mycotic hyphae and unidentified crystals in canine urine sediment. Unstained: high power magnification.

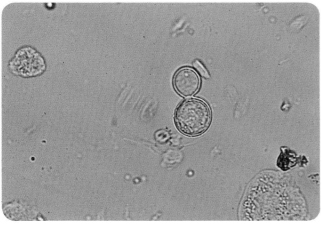

Fig. 62. Budding yeast form of blastomycosis. Unstained x 160 = original magnification.

2. SIGNIFICANCE

    a. Yeasts and fungi usually represent contaminants.

    b. Infections with *Candida albicans* may occur, especially in patients with resistant urinary tract infections that have been unsuccessfully treated with a variety of antimicrobial agents for prolonged periods.

    c. On occasion, fungi (blastomycosis, cryptococcosis, *etc.*) may be observed in the urine sediment of patients with polysystemic fungal disease which involves the urinary system (especially the kidneys).

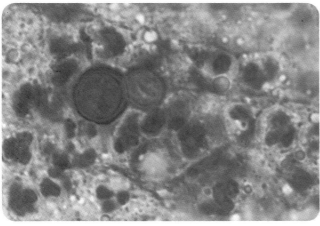

Fig. 63. Budding yeast form of blastomycosis surrounded by many white cells. New Methylene Blue stain: high power magnification.

1. APPEARANCE

    a. Yeasts have an ovoid shape, are colorless and often have characteristic budding forms. They are similar in size to RBC, but more variable.

    b. Fungi are usually characterized by distinct hyphae, which are often segmented.

    c. Occasionally characteristic forms of deep systemic mycotic agents (blastomycosis, cryptococcosis, *etc.*) may be detected in urine sediment.

H. PARASITES

1. DIOCTOPHYMA RENALE (Figure 64)

    a. Eggs of *D. renale* are thick-shelled, oval and have characteristic surface mammilations, except at their poles.

    b. Ova of *D. renale* may be observed in the urine sediment of animals (especially dogs) infected with this parasite, provided a gravid female is present in the excretory pathway of the urinary system.

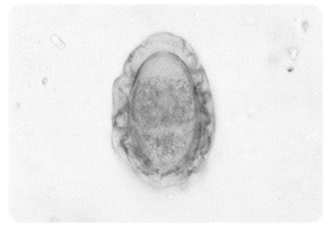

Fig. 64. *Dioctophyma renale* ovum. Unstained: high power magnification.

2. CAPILLARIA PLICA (Figure 65)

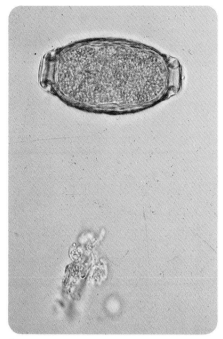

Fig. 65. *Capillaria plica* ovum. Unstained x 160 = original magnification.

a. Ova of *C. plica* are oval in shape and have bipolar plugs. They are colorless and have a slightly pitted shell.

b. Care must be used to differentiate the ova of *C. plica* from *Trichuris vulpus* ova that have appeared in urine as a result of fecal contamination.

3. MICROFILARIA OF DIROFILARIA IMMITIS (Figure 66)

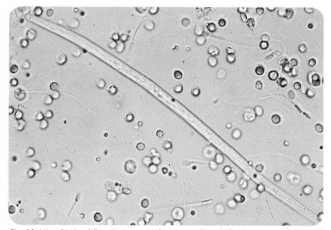

Fig. 66. Microfilaria of *Dirofilaria immitis* in urine sediment of a dog surrounded by red blood cells, white cells, spermatozoa and an occasional epithelial cell. Unstained x 40 = original magnification.

Microfilaria of *D. immitis* may occasionally be observed in the urine sediment of infected dogs, presumably as a result of hemorrhage into the excretory pathway of the urinary system.

I. SPERMATOZOA (Figures 67-68)

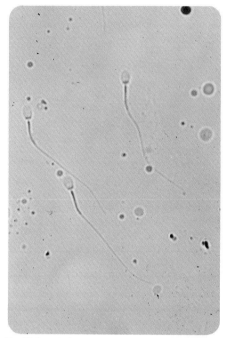

Fig. 67. Squad of spermatozoa surrounded by air bubbles. Unstained x 160 = original magnification.

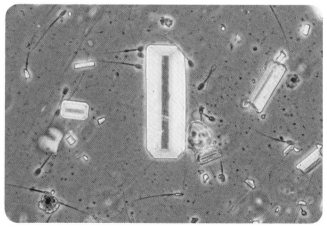

Fig. 68. Phosphate crystals and spermatozoa. Unstained phase microscopy x 102 = original magnification.

1. Spermatozoa are a normal finding in the urine of uncastrated male dogs and cats.

2. They may be readily identified by their characteristic shape.

3. They may be observed in bladder urine obtained by cystocentesis of male dogs, apparently as a result of reflux and/or their motility.

4. On occasion, sperm are present as a contaminant in the urine of females following breeding.

J. LIPIDURIA (Figure 69; *see* Figures 54 and 89).

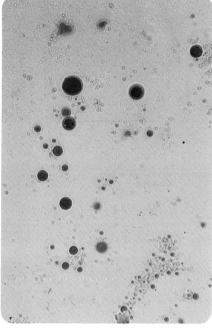

Fig. 69. Lipid droplets. Sudan IV stain x 40 = original magnification.

1. APPEARANCE

a. Under low magnification with subdued light, lipid droplets appear as black, refractile spheres of variable size. As they float to the undersurface of the coverslip, they may move out of the plane of focus of other heavier elements in the sediment.

b. They have an orange to red color when stained with Sudan III or IV (*see* Figure 69).

c. Lipid droplets that contain cholesterol typically have a "Maltese Cross" appearance when examined with the aid of polarization light microscopy.

2. SIGNIFICANCE

a. The origin of fat droplets is often difficult to determine.

b. Fat droplets may originate as a result of physiologic attrition of tubular epithelial cells (especially in cats),

and/or as a result of abnormal cytoplasmic degenerative changes in tubular epithelial cells.

c. Lipid-like droplets may occur as a result of contamination of urine with lubricants or the lining of some waterproof paper containers.

d. There is no apparent correlation between lipemia and lipiduria.

K. CRYSTALS (Figures 70-83; *see* Figure 68).

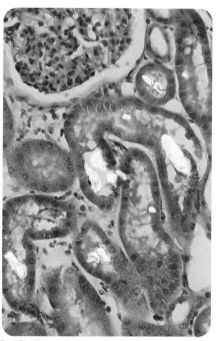

Fig. 70. Photomicrograph of ethylene glycol-induced oxalate crystals in the renal tubules of a dog. Hematoxylin and Eosin stain. Polarization microscopy x 160 = original magnification.

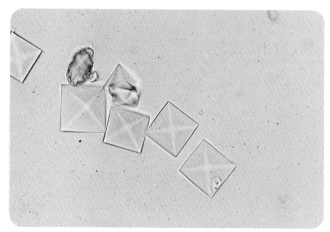

Fig. 71. Calcium oxalate dihydrate crystals. Unstained x 160 = original magnification.

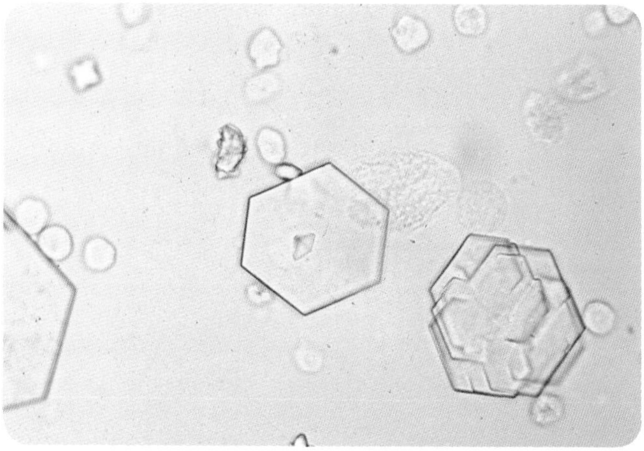

Fig. 72. Cystine crystals surrounded by white cells and occasional oxalate crystals and epithelial cells. Unstained x 100 = original magnification.

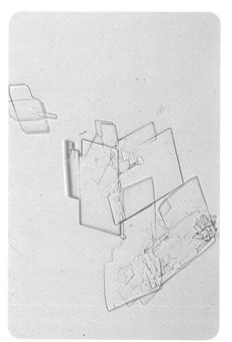

Fig. 73. Cholesterol crystals in canine urine sediment. Unstained x 100 = original magnification.

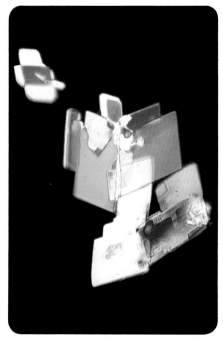

Fig. 74. Cholesterol crystals in canine urine sediment. Unstained polarizing light microscopy x 100 = original magnification.

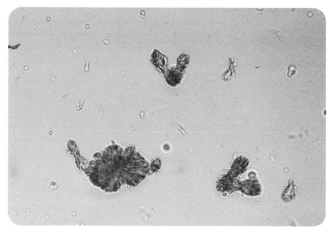

Fig. 75. Ammonium biurate (sometimes called ammonium urate) crystals. Unstained x 100 = original magnification.

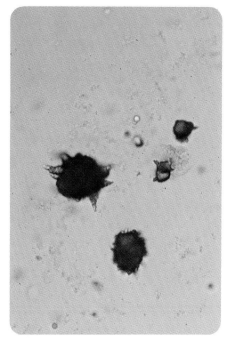

Fig. 76. Ammonium biurate crystals (thornapple form). Unstained x 160 = original magnification.

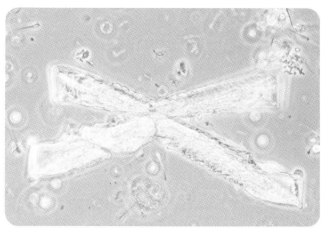

Fig. 77. Phosphate crystals. Unstained phase microscopy x 82 = original magnification.

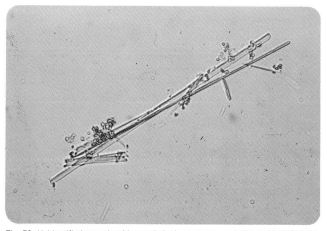

Fig. 79. Unidentified crystals with morphologic appearance similar to hippuric acid, calcium sulfate, and tyrosine crystals. Unstained x 160 = original magnification.

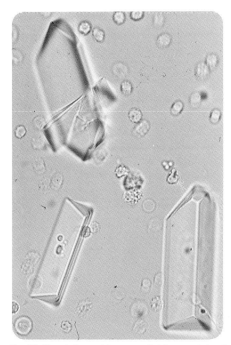

Fig. 78. Phosphate crystals surrounded by crenated red cells, an occasional white cell and occasional spermatozoa. Unstained x 100 = original magnification.

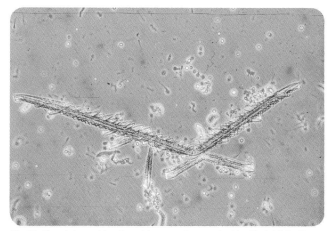

Fig. 80. Phosphate crystals adjacent to spermatozoa and unidentified debris; 40 x = original magnification.

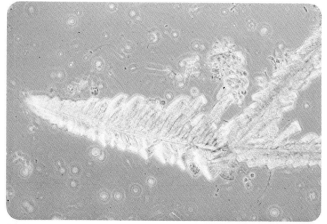

Fig. 81. Phosphate crystals. Unstained phase microscopy x 64 = original magnification.

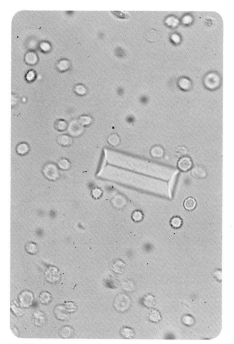

Fig. 82. Phosphate crystal, red cells, and white cells. Unstained x 160 = original magnification.

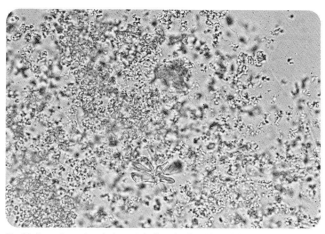

Fig. 83. Amorphous phosphate crystals. Unstained x 160 = original magnification.

1. Crystals in urine may be normal or abnormal; therefore, caution must be used in interpreting their significance.
2. In order to recognize abnormal crystals of clinical significance, one should be able to identify commonly-occurring crystals (Table 17).
3. Crystal formation is influenced by several variables including:

   a. Urine pH.

   b. Temperature.

   c. Solubility.

   d. Concentration of the crystalloid.

   e. Administration of medications.

Table 17

Characteristics of Urine Crystals

TYPE	DESCRIPTION	pH WHERE FOUND		
		ACID	NEUTRAL	ALKALINE
Cholesterol	Flat, colorless plates with corner notch	+	+	−
Calcium carbonate	Tiny, colorless spheres or dumbbells	−	+	+
Calcium oxalate	Small, colorless envelopes; sometimes dumbbell and ring forms	+	+	±
Cystine	Flat, colorless hexagonal plates	+	−	−
Leucine	Yellow spheres with radial striations	+	−	−
Phosphates (ammonium, magnesium)	3- to 6-sided colorless prisms	±	+	+
Phosphates (calcium)	Amorphous or long thin prisms	±	+	+
Tyrosine	Fine, colorless or yellow needles arranged in sheaves or rosettes	+	−	−
Urates (amorphous Ca, Mg, K)	Fine, yellow-red amorphous granules	+	−	−
Urates (ammonium)	Yellow-brown spheres (thornapples)	−	−	+

4. A fresh sample should be evaluated since *in vitro* changes in pH and temperature that occur following collection may change the spectrum of crystals observed. Ideally, fresh samples should be examined when they are at body temperature, rather than at room or refrigeration temperature.

5. Because many crystals are transparent and thin, it is advisable to examine urine sediment with reduced intensity of light.

6. The time and expense required to identify crystals on the basis of their reactions with chemicals and their X-ray diffraction properties are usually not worthwhile (cystine is an exception).

7. Cystine crystals have a characteristic hexagon (benzene ring) shape and are most often present in concentrated acid urine (*see* Figure 72). They are not normal constituents of urine, being associated with cystinuria.

8. Calcium oxalate dihydrate crystals have a characteristic octahedral or envelope shape (*see* Figures 70-72). They may be normal, occur in association with oxalate urolithiasis or occur in association with ethylene glycol toxicity (*see* Figure 70). Oxalate crystalluria is not a consistent finding, however, in patients intoxicated with ethylene glycol. When present, they may be in the form of calcium oxalate monohydrate.

9. Tyrosine and leucine crystals may indicate hepatic disease. (Figure 79).

10. Ammonium urate (ammonium biurate) crystals may be normal and have been commonly observed in dogs with portal vein anomalies (*see* Figures 75-76).

11. Struvite (magnesium ammonium phosphate) crystals may occur in normal dogs, in dogs with urinary tract infection associated with an alkaline urine pH, in dogs with struvite uroliths and in dogs with nonstruvite uroliths (*see* Figures 68, 77-83).

12. On occasion, excretion of drugs may result in formation of urine crystals. Sulfonamides, ampicillin and radiopaque contrast material may on occasion form crystals in urine.

   a. Because of the solubility characteristics of sulfonamide drugs currently used, and the decreased frequency with which sulfonamides are used because of availability of superior antimicrobial agents, sulfonamide crystalluria has become relatively uncommon. Sulfonamide crystals are typically yellow-brown asymmetrical crystals grouped in sheaves or rosettes.

   b. Radiopaque contrast media have been reported to produce long, thin rectangles of flat, four-sided, notched plates in human beings.

   c. Ampicillin has been reported to produce long, thin, clear crystals in man.

L. ARTIFACTS AND CONTAMINANTS (Figures 84-90; *see* Figure 68)

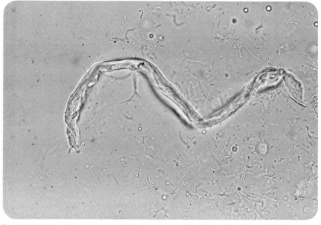

Fig. 84. Cotton fiber surrounded by numerous bacteria. Unstained: high power magnification.

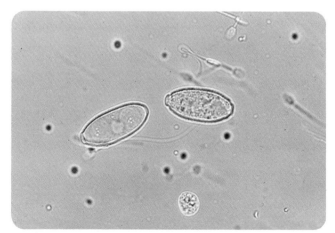

Fig. 85. Pollen grains and sperm. Unstained x 160 = original magnification.

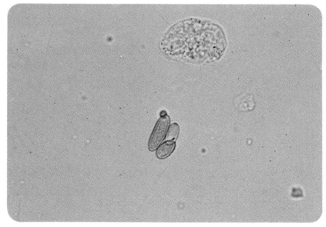

Fig. 86. Pollen grains. Unstained x 160 = original magnification.

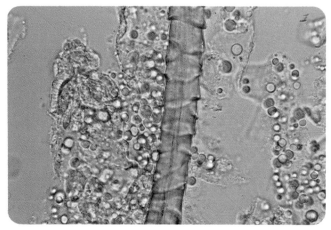

Fig. 89. Hair shaft surrounded by lipid droplets and debris. Unstained: low power magnification.

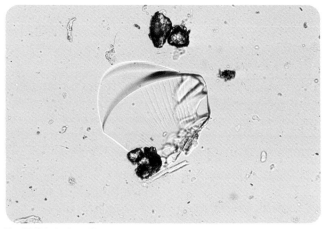

Fig. 87. Chip in glass slide. Unstained: low power magnification.

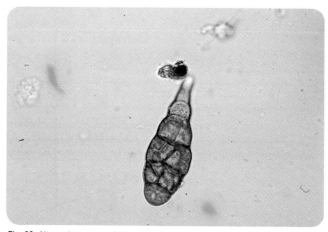

Fig. 90. Alternaria, a contaminant of urine. Unstained x 160 = original magnification.

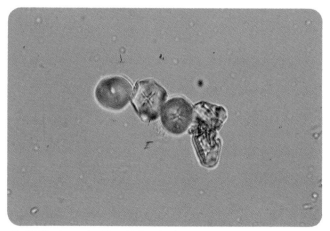

Fig. 88. Starch granules (Biosorb). Unstained x 64 = original magnification.

1. Many exogenous substances may contaminate urine and are a potential source of confusion.
2. Commonly encountered artifacts and contaminants include air bubbles (*see* Figure 68), oil droplets from lubricants, starch granules from surgical gloves (*see* Figure 88), glass particles and chips in glass slides (*see* Figure 87), hair (*see* Figure 89), fecal material (including parasite ova), bacteria and yeasts or fungi, dust, fragments of cotton or other fabrics (*see* Figure 84), and plant spores (*see* Figures 85, 86, and 90).

Chapter 9. Interpretation of Clinical Cases

Interpretation of Clinical Cases

CASE 1

Consider the following results obtained by analysis of a noncatheterized urine sample from an 8-year-old male Dachshund:

TEST	RESULTS	TEST	RESULTS
Color	Yellow	Protein	1+
Turbidity	Cloudy	RBC	10-15/HPF
Specific gravity	1.039	WBC	5-10/HPF
pH	6.5	Casts	Many granular/LPF
Glucose	Negative	Epithelial cells	Moderate
Acetone	Negative	Bacteria	None
Bilirubin	Negative	Crystals	Occasional oxalate
Occult blood	1+		

The best interpretation of the results of this urinalysis is that the patient:

a. *Has acute primary renal failure.*

b. *Has chronic primary renal failure.*

c. *Has acute renal disease.*

d. *Has chronic renal disease.*

e. *Is normal.*

ANSWER = c

COMMENTS:

a. Concentration of urine to this degree indicates that an adequate population of nephrons is functional to prevent primary renal failure. The small quantity of protein and high specific gravity indicate that primary renal failure and glomerulotubular imbalance are improbable.

b. See comment a.

c. Detection of many granular casts is indicative of renal disease, even though urine concentration indicates that the disease is not of sufficient magnitude to cause renal failure. The large number of casts suggests (but does not prove) that the disorder is acute.

d. This answer is possible, although c is more probable. Additional information would be required to prove or disprove either answer.

e. The findings are definitely abnormal.

CASE 2

Consider the following results obtained by analysis of a fresh urine sample obtained by catheterization:

TEST	RESULTS	TEST	RESULTS
Color	Yellow	Protein	2+
Turbidity	Cloudy	RBC	Numerous/HPF
Specific gravity	1.040	WBC	Numerous/HPF
pH	8.0	Casts	None
Glucose	Negative	Epithelial cells	Many
Acetone	Negative	Bacteria	Many rods
Bilirubin	Negative	Crystals	Moderate phosphate
Occult blood	4+		

The best interpretation of the results of this urinalysis is that the patient:

a. Has an inflammatory process somewhere along the urinary tract caused by bacterial infection.

b. Has an inflammatory process somewhere along the genitourinary tract caused by bacterial infection.

c. Has an inflammatory process somewhere along the urinary tract caused or complicated by bacterial infection.

d. Is normal, and that the sample was contaminated during the process of analysis.

e. Has struvite uroliths associated with urinary tract infection.

ANSWER = c

COMMENTS:

a. The results do not permit differentiation between bacterial infection as a cause or complication of urinary tract infection.

b. Although this answer is not totally incorrect, to conclude definitely that the genital tract is involved in a sample obtained by catheterization is an overstatement.

c. In light of comments a and b, this appears to be the best interpretation.

d. The results are definitely abnormal and would not be expected to be caused by contamination.

e. Although magnesium ammonium phosphate uroliths may be present, phosphate crystalluria is not a reliable index of their occurrence. Phosphate crystals may be normal or abnormal.

CASE 3

A five-year-old female Cocker Spaniel is admitted as an emergency to your hospital in the late hours of the evening because of severe vomiting. The owner has no information about the dog's urination habits. Physical examination reveals that the dog is dehydrated (9% loss of body weight due to fluid); an appropriate quantity of lactated Ringer's solution is administered parenterally to correct the dehydration. The next morning samples of urine and blood are collected for analysis. Consider the following results:

URINALYSIS

TEST	RESULTS	TEST	RESULTS
Color	Light Yellow	Protein	Negative
Turbidity	Clear	RBC	Occasional
Specific gravity	1.014	WBC	Occasional
pH	5.5	Casts	None
Glucose	Negative	Epithelial cells	Many
Acetone	Negative	Bacteria	Negative
Bilirubin	Negative	Crystals	Few amorphous crystals

ADDITIONAL LABORATORY DATA

TEST	RESULTS
Blood urea nitrogen	65 mg/100 ml
Serum amylase	Two times normal value
Hemogram: PCV = 49	
WBC = 23,000	
Total neutrophils = 80% (75% mature, 5% immature)	
Lymphocytes = 10%	
Monocytes = 10%	

The best interpretation of these findings is that:

a. *The dog has prerenal azotemia caused by fluid loss due to vomiting.*

b. *The dog has primary renal failure associated with an impaired ability to concentrate urine, azotemia, vomiting and dehydration.*

c. *The dog has hypoadrenocorticism associated with vomiting, impaired renal conservation of sodium and water and prerenal azotemia.*

d. *The dog has azotemia but no inference about cause can be established with this data.*

e. *The dog has acute pancreatitis associated with concomitant primary renal failure.*

ANSWER = d
COMMENTS:

a. Although a prerenal cause of azotemia is possible, failure to collect a urine sample prior to parenteral fluid administration precludes determination of whether the low urine specific gravity was induced by diuresis or impaired ability of the kidneys to concentrate urine.

b. This situation is possible but cannot be confirmed because parenteral fluids were given prior to collection of a urine sample (see a).

c. See comments a and b.

d. See comments a and b.

e. See comments a and b.

CASE 4

Consider the following results obtained by analysis of a non-catheterized urine sample from a 3-year-old male Collie:

TEST	RESULTS	TEST	RESULTS
Color	Yellow	Protein	1+
Turbidity	Cloudy	RBC	0-1/HPF
Specific gravity	1.050	WBC	0-1/HPF
pH	7.5	Casts	None
Glucose	Negative	Epithelial cells	Occasional
Acetone	Negative	Bacteria	None
Bilirubin	Negative	Crystals	Many phosphate
Occult blood	Negative		

The best interpretation of the significance of the proteinuria is that it is:

a. *Clinically insignificant.*

b. *Indicative of generalized glomerular disease.*

c. *Indicative of generalized tubular disease.*

d. *Indicative of damage to the transitional epithelium lining the urinary tract.*

e. *Indicative of nonurinary proteinuria.*

ANSWER = *a*

COMMENTS:

a. Detection of slight proteinuria in highly concentrated urine is a common finding in dogs.

b. This is a possibility, but would require additional studies to prove.

c. This is a possibility, but unlikely in light of other findings.

d. This problem would be expected to be associated with an inflammatory response, hematuria and/or many transitional epithelial cells.

e. Further information would be required to verify this conclusion.

CASE 5

A 5-year-old female Toy Collie is admitted to your hospital because of progressive vomiting, polydipsia and lethargy of at least three days' duration. The frequency and volume of the dog's micturition were not observed by the owner. Physical examination reveals that the rate and character of the dog's pulse and respiration are normal. The rectal temperature is 103.5° F. The dog is clinically (8%) dehydrated. The following laboratory data are obtained:

HEMOGRAM

TEST	RESULTS	TEST	RESULTS
PCV	57%	Stabs	27%
Total WBC	27,000/cmm	Monocytes	8%
Segmenters	60%	Lymphocytes	5%

ADDITIONAL LABORATORY DATA

TEST	RESULTS
Specific gravity	1.035
Protein	Trace
Blood urea nitrogen	90 mg/100 ml
Serum amylase	Elevated (4 times normal value)

Which of the following conclusions is most probable? This dog has:

a. *Pancreatitis.*

b. *Primary renal failure.*

c. *Pancreatitis and primary renal failure.*

d. *Pancreatitis and prerenal azotemia*

e. *Hypoadrenocorticism.*

ANSWER = *d*

COMMENTS:

a. Although the findings support a diagnosis of pancreatitis, they do not provide an explanation of the azotemia.

b. Ability to concentrate urine to this degree indicates that a sufficient population of functional nephrons is present to prevent signs of primary renal failure.

c. See comment b.

d. Loss of fluid caused by vomiting secondary to acute pancreatitis is commonly associated with prerenal azotemia.

e. Although this disorder is a possibility, acute pancreatitis and prerenal azotemia is a probability.

CASE 6

Consider the following results obtained by analysis of a non-catheterized urine sample:

TEST	RESULTS	TEST	RESULTS
Color	Light yellow	Protein	4+
Turbidity	Clear	RBC	0-1/HPF
Specific gravity	1.035	WBC	1-2/HPF
pH	6.5	Casts	Occasional hyaline
Glucose	Negative	Epithelial cells	Occasional
Acetone	Negative	Bacteria	None
Bilirubin	Negative	Crystals	None
Occult blood	Negative		

The best interpretation of the results of this urinalysis is that the patient:

a. Is normal.

b. Has generalized glomerular disease.

c. Has an inflammatory process somewhere along the urinary tract.

d. Has generalized tubular disease.

e. Has findings indicative of congestive heart failure or fever.

ANSWER = b

COMMENTS:

a. Proteinuria of this magnitude is not normal.

b. Marked proteinuria in the absence of significant numbers of red blood cells and white cells is the hallmark of generalized glomerular disease in dogs and cats.

c. Absence of significant numbers of red blood cells and white cells eliminates an inflammatory response.

d. Proteinuria of this magnitude would not be expected as a result of primary tubular disease.

e. Proteinuria of this magnitude would not be expected as a result of nonurinary causes of proteinuria.

CASE 7

Consider the following results obtained by analysis of a noncatheterized urine sample:

TEST	RESULTS	TEST	RESULTS
Color	Light yellow	Protein	Negative
Turbidity	Clear	RBC	Negative
Specific gravity	1.002	WBC	Negative
pH	6.0	Casts	None
Glucose	Negative	Epithelial cells	None
Bilirubin	Negative	Bacteria	None
Acetone	Negative		
Occult blood	Negative		

The best interpretation of the results of this urinalysis is that:

a. *There is an insufficient population of viable nephrons to concentrate glomerular filtrate.*

b. *There is a sufficient population of viable nephrons to dilute glomerular filtrate.*

c. *There is a sufficient population of nephrons to concentrate or dilute glomerular filtrate.*

d. *All of the nephrons of both kidneys are functional.*

e. *More than 2/3 of the nephrons of both kidneys are nonfunctional.*

ANSWER = *b*

COMMENTS:

a. This conclusion could not be established without knowledge of the patient's hydration status, a water-deprivation test and perhaps a vasopressin response test. The fact that urine dilution of this magnitude has occurred suggests that a sufficient population of functional nephrons is present to concentrate urine.

b. Dilution of glomerular filtrate to this degree requires a sufficient population of functional nephrons (at least $\frac{1}{3}$ in dogs) to remove solute in excess of water.

c. See comment a.

d. It is not possible to evaluate the functional status of all nephrons on the basis of urine specific gravity. Many nephrons may be nonfunctional (up to $\frac{2}{3}$ in dogs and probably more in cats) without loss of the ability to concentrate urine, at least to some degree.

e. See comment b.

CASE 8

Consider the following results obtained by analysis of a non-catheterized urine sample from an 8-year-old female Pug:

TEST	RESULTS	TEST	RESULTS
Color	Yellow	Protein	Trace
Turbidity	Clear	RBC	1-3/HPF
Specific gravity	1.058	WBC	0-1/HPF
pH	6.5	Casts	None
Glucose	Negative	Epithelial cells	Occasional
Acetone	Negative	Bacteria	None
Bilirubin	1+	Crystals	Amorphous debris
Occult blood	Negative		

The best interpretation of the results of this urinalysis is that the patient:

a. Has hepatic disease.

b. Has an inflammatory disease syndrome of the urinary tract.

c. Is normal.

d. Has acute renal failure.

e. Has slight injury to the glomeruli.

ANSWER = c
COMMENTS:

a. A mild degree of bilirubinuria in highly concentrated dog urine is often a normal finding. Bilirubinuria of any magnitude is usually indicative of some underlying disease in cats, however.

b. Proteinuria, hematuria and pyuria of this magnitude are normal findings, especially in highly concentrated urine.

c. See comment a.

d. Concentration of urine to this degree precludes a diagnosis of primary renal failure.

e. Proteinuria of this magnitude in highly concentrated urine is not indicative of glomerular disease.

CASE 9

Consider the following results obtained by analysis of a non-catheterized urine sample:

TEST	RESULTS	TEST	RESULTS
Color	Light yellow	Protein	2+
Turbidity	Slightly cloudy	RBC	25-30/HPF
Specific gravity	1.011	WBC	60-70/HPF
pH	5.5	Casts	Occasional WBC/HPF
Glucose	Negative	Epithelial cells	Moderate
Acetone	Negative	Bacteria	Rods
Bilirubin	Negative	Crystals	None
Occult blood	1+		

The best interpretation of this urinalysis is that the patient has an infectious inflammatory disease involving at least the:

a. Urinary tract.

b. Urinary bladder.

c. Renal tubules.

d. Glomeruli.

e. Renal vessels.

ANSWER = c

COMMENTS:

a. Detection of white cell casts permits localization beyond the urinary tract.

b. See comment a.

c. Detection of WBC casts is reliable evidence of tubular involvement in the infectious inflammatory process.

d. Available data do not permit confirmation or elimination of glomerular involvement.

e. Available data do not permit confirmation or elimination of renal vascular involvement.

CASE 10

Consider the following results obtained by urinalysis of a noncatheterized urine sample:

TEST	RESULTS	TEST	RESULTS
Color	Yellow	Protein	Negative
Turbidity	Clear	RBC	Negative
Specific gravity	1.012	WBC	Negative
pH	6.5	Casts	Negative
Glucose	Negative	Epithelial cells	Negative
Acetone	Negative	Bacteria	Negative
Bilirubin	Negative	Crystals	Few phosphate
Occult blood	Negative		

The best interpretation of the results of this urinalysis is that:

a. The patient's kidneys have lost the ability to concentrate and dilute urine.

b. The patient's kidneys have lost the ability to concentrate urine.

c. The patient's kidneys have lost the ability to dilute urine.

d. No conclusions can be established about the ability of the patient's kidneys to concentrate and dilute urine.

e. The patient has a fixed urine specific gravity, probably as a result of primary renal failure.

ANSWER = d

COMMENTS:

a. Since a urine specific gravity may represent a normal or abnormal value, further information must be obtained before renal concentrating and diluting capacity can be assessed.

b. See comment a.

c. See comment a.

d. See comment a.

e. See comment a.

CASE 11

Consider the following results obtained by analysis of a noncatheterized urine sample obtained from a cat:

TEST	RESULTS	TEST	RESULTS
Color	Yellow	Protein	Trace
Turbidity	Clear	RBC	1-3/HPF
Specific gravity	1.050	WBC	0-1/HPF
pH	6.5	Casts	None
Glucose	Negative	Epithelial cells	Occasional
Acetone	Negative	Bacteria	None
Bilirubin	1+	Crystals	Amorphous phosphates
Occult blood	Negative		

The best interpretation of the results of this urinalysis is that the patient:

a. *Has significant bilirubinuria.*

b. *Has inflammatory disease syndrome along the urinary tract.*

c. *Is normal.*

d. *Has acute renal failure.*

e. *Has lower urinary tract disease.*

ANSWER = a

COMMENTS:

a. Unlike dogs, bilirubinuria in cats, even when present in small quantities in concentrated urine, is usually indicative of an underlying disorder.

b. Hematuria and pyuria of this magnitude in concentrated urine is usually a normal finding.

c. See comment a.

d. The capacity to concentrate urine to this degree precludes a diagnosis of primary renal failure.

e. See comment b.

CASE 12

A 5-year-old, obese, nonspayed, female German Shepherd dog is admitted to your hospital with intermittent hematuria which has not yet responded to continuous therapy with ampicillin. The owners have observed that the blood is voided throughout micturition. Physical examination reveals no abnormalities but abdominal palpation is difficult because of the obese nature of the dog. Consider the following results:

URINALYSIS

TEST	RESULTS	TEST	RESULTS
Color	Reddish brown	Protein	2+
Turbidity	Cloudy	RBC	Many
Specific gravity	1.020	WBC	Many
pH	7.5	Casts	None
Glucose	Negative	Epithelial cells	Many
Acetone	Negative	Bacteria	None
Bilirubin	Negative	Crystals	Many triple phosphate
Occult blood	3+		

Urine Culture for Aerobic Bacteria: Sterile

The best interpretation of these findings is that the:

a. *Cause and location of the hematuria cannot be established.*

b. *Hematuria has originated from the kidneys, but the cause is unknown.*

c. *Hematuria has originated from the kidneys, and is probably caused by a calculus or neoplasm.*

d. *Hematuria has been caused by an anaerobic bacteria or virus.*

e. *The dog has cystitis caused by a diverticulum of the bladder wall.*

ANSWER = *a*
COMMENTS:

a. Additional information is required to localize the source of hematuria.

b. Hematuria throughout micturition can originate from any location within the urinary system.

c. See comment b.

d. These are possibilities but have not been confirmed.

e. See comment a.

CASE 13

Consider the following results obtained by analysis of a non-catheterized urine sample:

TEST	RESULTS	TEST	RESULTS
Color	Yellow	Protein	2+
Turbidity	Cloudy	RBC	50-60/HPF
Specific gravity	1.024	WBC	Numerous/ HPF
pH	6.5	Casts	Occasional casts
Glucose	Negative	Epithelial cells	Many
Acetone	Negative	Bacteria	None
Bilirubin	Negative	Crystals	None
Occult blood	2+		

The best interpretation of the results of this urinalysis is that the patient has:

a. *Infection somewhere in the urinary tract.*

b. *Infection somewhere in the genitourinary system.*

c. *Inflammation somewhere in the urinary tract.*

d. *Inflammation somewhere in the genitourinary system.*

e. *Inflammation involving the renal tubules.*

ANSWER = *d*
COMMENTS:

a. The fact that the inflammatory response has been caused or complicated by an infection has not been established.

b. See comment a.

c. Collection of a voided urine sample does not exclude the genital tract from consideration.

d. The inflammatory components in this sample could have originated in the urinary and/or genital system.

e. This data is not sufficiently specific to localize the inflammatory process to the renal tubules.

CASE 14

Consider the following results obtained by analysis of a non-catheterized urine sample:

TEST	RESULTS	TEST	RESULTS
Color	Yellow	Protein	Trace
Turbidity	Clear	RBC	1-3/HPF
Specific gravity	1.029	WBC	0-1/HPF
pH	7.0	Casts	None
Glucose	Negative	Epithelial cells	Occasional
Acetone	Negative	Bacteria	None
Bilirubin	Negative	Crystals	Ammonium urate
Occult blood	Negative		

The best interpretation of the results of this urinalysis is that the patient:

a. *Has hepatic disease.*

b. *Has inflammatory disease syndrome along the urinary tract.*

c. *Is normal.*

d. *Has acute renal failure.*

e. *Has urate uroliths.*

ANSWER = *c*
COMMENTS:

a. Although ammonium urate crystals have been reported in dogs with hepatic vascular anomalies, they are not a consistent finding in these disorders nor pathognomonic of these disorders.

b. The degree of proteinuria, pyuria and hematuria is not indicative of inflammation.

c. All findings in this sample are compatible with normalcy.

d. Concentration of urine excludes renal failure as a diagnostic probability.

e. Ammonium urate crystals are not a reliable index of ammonium urate uroliths since they may occur normally and they may occur in association with disorders without urate uroliths.

CASE 15

Consider the following results obtained by analysis of a noncatheterized urine sample:

TEST	RESULTS	TEST	RESULTS
Color	Yellow/ orange	Protein	Trace
Turbidity	Cloudy	RBC	None
Specific gravity	1.027	WBC	0-1/HPF
pH	7.0	Casts	None
Glucose	Negative	Epithelial cells	Occasional
Acetone	Negative	Bacteria	None
Bilirubin	3+	Crystals	Occasional phosphate
Occult blood	Negative		

The best interpretation of the results of this urinalysis is that the patient:

a. Is normal.

b. Probably has obstructive or hepatocellular liver disease.

c. Probably has hemolytic jaundice.

d. Probably has generalized glomerular disease.

e. Probably has phosphate calculi.

ANSWER = *b*
COMMENTS:

a. Bilirubinuria of this magnitude is not normal.

b. Bilirubinuria of this magnitude is usually associated with hepatocellular or obstructive liver diseases.

c. Hemolytic jaundice may be associated with bilirubinuria, but also is typically associated with a positive occult blood test.

d. Proteinuria of this magnitude is not indicative of significant alteration of glomerular capillary permeability.

e. Phosphate crystalluria is not a reliable index of calcium phosphate or magnesium ammonium phosphate calculi.

CASE 16

Consider the following results obtained by analysis of a catheterized urine sample:

TEST	RESULTS	TEST	RESULTS
Color	Yellow	Protein	2+
Turbidity	Slightly cloudy	RBC	Numerous/ HPF
Specific gravity	1.027	WBC	1-3/HPF
pH	7.0	Casts	None
Glucose	Negative	Epithelial cells	Occasional
Acetone	Negative	Bacteria	None
Bilirubin	Negative	Crystals	Many phosphate
Occult blood	3+		

The best interpretation of the results of this urinalysis is that the patient has:

a. Iatrogenic hematuria induced by rough catheterization.

b. An inflammatory disease of the urinary tract.

c. Hematuria induced by phosphate calculi.

d. Pyelonephritis.

e. Hemorrhage of the urinary tract excluding the urethra.

ANSWER = a
COMMENTS:

a. Traumatic hemorrhage induced with urinary catheters commonly is associated with hematuria and proteinuria. Proteinuria is primarily caused by loss of plasma proteins with RBC in whole blood.

b. The paucity of white cells compared to red blood cells is not indicative of an inflammatory response.

c. Phosphate crystalluria is not a reliable index of calcium phosphate or magnesium ammonium phosphate calculi. In addition, phosphate calculi are commonly associated with an infectious inflammatory response.

d. The findings are not indicative of renal involvement in an inflammatory process.

e. The urethra cannot be excluded as a source of hemorrhage just because the sample was obtained by catheterization.

CASE 17

Consider the following results obtained by analysis of a non-catheterized urine sample:

TEST	RESULTS	TEST	RESULTS
Color	Yellow	Protein	Negative
Turbidity	Cloudy	RBC	Negative
Specific gravity	1.025	WBC	Negative
pH	8.0	Casts	Negative
Glucose	Negative	Epithelial cells	Occasional
Acetone	Negative	Bacteria	Many rods and cocci
Bilirubin	Negative	Crystals	Many phosphate
Occult blood	Negative		

The best interpretation of the results of this urinalysis is that:

a. *The sample was collected in a nonsterilized container and was analyzed several hours following collection.*

b. *The patient has an infectious inflammatory disease of the urinary bladder.*

c. *The patient has an infectious inflammatory disease of the genital or urinary tract.*

d. *The urine sample has been contaminated with bacteria located in the genital tract.*

e. *The patient has phosphate calculi associated with urinary tract infection.*

ANSWER = *a*

COMMENTS:

a. Proliferation of urease-producing bacteria following collection would account for significant bacteriuria in absence of inflammatory components and alkalinization of the sample.

b. There are no signs of inflammation in the sample.

c. See comment b.

d. Although this is a possibility, one would also expect contamination with inflammatory cells.

e. Phosphate crystalluria is not a reliable index of calcium phosphate or magnesium ammonium phosphate calculi.

CASE 18

Consider the following results obtained by analysis of a catheterized urine sample:

TEST	RESULTS	TEST	RESULTS
Color	Yellow	Protein	2+
Turbidity	Cloudy	RBC	200/HPF
Specific gravity	1.035	WBC	200/HPF
pH	8.5	Casts	None
Glucose	Negative	Epithelial cells	Occasional
Acetone	Negative	Bacteria	Rods
Bilirubin	Negative	Crystals	Many phosphates
Occult blood	4+		

The best interpretation of the results of this urinalysis is that the patient:

a. *Has cystic calculi caused by bacterial infection.*

b. *Has a primary bacterial infection of the urinary bladder.*

c. *Has a secondary bacterial infection of the urinary bladder.*

d. *Has inflammatory disease of the urinary tract caused or complicated by bacterial infection.*

e. *Has iatrogenic hematuria caused by catheterization.*

ANSWER = d
COMMENTS:

a. Phosphate crystalluria is not a reliable index of calcium phosphate or magnesium ammonium phosphate calculi.

b. Collection of urine by catheterization will not permit localization of an infectious inflammatory response to the urinary bladder.

c. See comment b.

d. The inflammatory response may have been caused or complicated by bacterial infection. It involves at least the bladder, ureters, and/or kidneys. Urethral involvement, however, cannot be ruled out.

e. The findings indicate an infectious inflammatory response rather than hematuria.

CASE 19

Consider the following results obtained by analysis of a non-catheterized urine sample:

TEST	RESULTS	TEST	RESULTS
Color	Yellow	Protein	1+
Turbidity	Cloudy	RBC	None
Specific gravity	1.005	WBC	None
pH	6.5	Casts	None
Glucose	None	Epithelial cells	Many
Acetone	None	Bacteria	None
Bilirubin	None	Crystals	None
Occult blood	4+		

The best interpretation of the significance of the positive occult blood test is that it was caused by:

a. *Red blood cells.*

b. *Red blood cells or hemoglobin.*

c. *Red blood cells, hemoglobin or myoglobin.*

d. *A drug administered to the patient.*

e. *Red blood cells or myoglobin.*

ANSWER = c

COMMENTS:

a. A positive chemical test of this magnitude may be indicative of hematuria, hemoglobinuria or myoglobinuria. Absence of RBC from the urine sediment might have occurred as a result of hemolysis in a very dilute urine sample.

b. See comment a.

c. See comment a.

d. Excretion of drugs that cause a false positive reaction is an extremely unlikely cause of the positive occult blood test.

e. See comment a.

CASE 20

Consider the following results obtained by analysis of a non-catheterized urine sample obtained from a 3-year-old Dachshund:

TEST	RESULTS	TEST	RESULTS
Color	Yellow	Protein	Trace
Turbidity	Clear	RBC	1-3/HPF
Specific gravity	1.048	WBC	0-1/HPF
pH	6.0	Casts	None
Glucose	Negative	Epithelial cells	Occasional
Acetone	Negative	Bacteria	None
Bilirubin	1+	Crystals	Cystine
Occult blood	Negative		

The best interpretation of the results of this urinalysis is that the patient:

a. Has hepatic disease.

b. Has inflammatory disease syndrome along the urinary tract.

c. Is normal.

d. Has acute renal failure.

e. Has cystinuria.

ANSWER = e
COMMENTS:

a. Bilirubinuria of this magnitude in concentrated canine urine is usually an insignificant finding.

b. Hematuria, pyuria and proteinuria of this magnitude in a concentrated urine sample is usually an insignificant finding.

c. Cystine crystals are not a normal component of urine.

d. Concentration of urine to this degree excludes renal failure as a diagnostic probability.

e. Cystine crystals are indicative of cystinuria. Cystinuria may occur in the absence of detectable cystine crystals, however, especially if the urine sample is alkaline and dilute.

CASE 21

Consider the following results obtained by analysis of a noncatheterized urine sample:

TEST	RESULTS	TEST	RESULTS
Color	Yellow	Protein	Negative
Turbidity	Cloudy	RBC	Negative
Specific gravity	1.032	WBC	Negative
pH	8.0	Casts	Negative
Glucose	Negative	Epithelial cells	Occasional
Acetone	Negative	Bacteria	Negative
Bilirubin	Negative	Crystals	Numerous phosphate
Occult blood	Negative		

The best interpretation of the results of this urinalysis is that the patient:

a. Has cystitis.

b. Has a urinary tract infection.

c. Is normal.

d. May have phosphate calculi.

e. Has metabolic alkalosis.

ANSWER = c
COMMENTS:

a. There is no evidence of inflammation in the urine sample.

b. There is no evidence of infection in the urine sample.

c. Although normal dog and cat urine is typically acidic, it can be alkaline. This is the most probable explanation.

d. Phosphate crystalluria and urine alkalinity are not a reliable index of calcium phosphate or magnesium ammonium phosphate uroliths.

e. Although metabolic alkalosis is a possibility, it is not probable. Additional information would be required to confirm this disorder.

CASE 22

Consider the following results obtained by analysis of a non-catheterized urine sample:

TEST	RESULTS	TEST	RESULTS
Color	Yellow	Protein	Negative
Turbidity	Slightly cloudy	RBC	0-1/HPF
Specific gravity	1.018	WBC	1-2/HPF
pH	6.0	Casts	None
Glucose	3+	Epithelial cells	Moderate
Acetone	Negative	Bacteria	Negative
Bilirubin	Negative	Crystals	Negative
Occult blood	Negative		

The best interpretation of the results of this urinalysis is that:

a. *The patient has diabetes mellitus.*

b. *The patient has glucosuria.*

c. *The patient has primary renal glucosuria.*

d. *The patient has the Fanconi syndrome.*

e. *The patient has generalized tubular disease.*

ANSWER = *b*
COMMENTS:

a. Glucosuria is not diagnostic of diabetes mellitus.

b. Glucosuria is not a normal finding in urine.

c. Glucosuria is not diagnostic of primary renal glucosuria.

d. Glucosuria may occur in association with the Fanconi syndrome, diabetes mellitus, primary renal glucosuria, and many other syndromes.

e. Glucosuria may occur in association with tubular dysfunction but it is not diagnostic of such a problem.

Appendix:
Selected Supplemental Bibliography
General References

Anonymous. (1974). *A Handbook of Kidney Nomenclature and Nosology.* Publ. Little, Brown & Co., Boston, MA.

Benjamin, M. M. (1978). *Outline of Veterinary Clinical Pathology (3rd Edition).* Publ. Iowa State University Press, Ames, IA.

Bradley, G. M. and Benson, E. S. (1974). Examination of the Urine. In: *Todd-Sanford Clinical Diagnosis by Laboratory Methods (15th Edition.)* Davidson, I., and Henry, J. B.)Ed.). Publ. W. B. Saunders, Philadelphia, PA.

Brody, L. H., Salladay, J. R., and Armbruster, K. (1971). Urinalysis and the Urinary Sediment. Med. Clin. North Am., *55:* 243-266.

Coles, E. H. (1974). *Veterinary Clinical Pathology (2nd Edition).* Publ. W. B. Saunders Co., Philadelphia, PA.

Duncan, J. R., and Prasse, K. W. (1976). Clinical Examination of the Urine. Vet. Clin. North Am., *6:* 647.

Duncan, J. R., and Prasse, K. W. (1977). *Veterinary Laboratory Medicine.* Publ. Iowa State University Press, Ames, IA.

Friedman, S. A., and Gladstone, J. L. (1971). The Effects of Hydration and Bladder Incubation Time on Urine Colony Counts. J. Urol., *105:* 428-432.

Hansten, P. D. (1975). *Drug Interactions (3rd Edition).* Publ. Lea & Febiger, Philadelphia, PA.

Henry, R.J. (1974). *Clinical Chemistry: Principles and Techniques.* Publ. Harper & Row, New York, NY.

Hindman, R., Tronic, B., and Bartlett, R. (1976). Effect of Delay on Culture of Urine. J. Clin. Microbiol., *4:* 102-107.

Hubert, W. T. (1972). Bacteria and Spermatozoa in the Canine Urinary Bladder. Cornell Vet., *62:* 13-20.

Kankeko, J.J. (1980). *Clinical Biochemistry of Domestic Animals, (3rd Edition).* Publ. Academic Press, New York, NY.

Kark, R. M., Lowrence, J. R., Pollak, V. E., Pirani, C. L., Muehrcke, R. C., and Silva, H. (1963). *A Primer of Urinalysis (2nd Edition).* Publ. Harper & Row, New York, NY.

Kurtaman, N. A., and Rogers, P. W. (1974). *A Handbook of Urinalysis and Urine Sediment.* Publ. Charles C. Thomas, Springfield, IL.

Kutter, D. (1977). *Rapid Clinical Diagnostic Tests.* Publ. Urban & Schwarzenberg, Baltimore, MD.

Leach, C. S., Rambault, P. C., and Fischer, C. L. (1975). A Comparative Study of Two Methods of Urine Preservation. Clin. Biochem., *8:* 108-117.

Lippman, R. W. (1957). *Urine and the Urinary Sediment.* Publ. Charles C. Thomas, Springfield, IL.

Osborne, C. A. (1970). Urologic Logic—Diagnosis of Renal Disease. JAVMA, *157:* 1656-1666.

Osborne, C. A., Low, D. G., and Finco, D. R. (169). Reversible versus Irreversible Renal Disease in the Dog. JAVMA, *155:* 2062-2078.

Osborne, C. A., Low, D. G., and Finco, D. R. (1982). *Canine and Feline Urology. (® 2nd Edition in preparation).* Publ. W. B. Saunders Co., Philadephia, PA.

Peele, H. D., Gadsen, R. H., and Crews, R. (1977). Semi-automated versus Visual Reading of Urinalysis Dipsticks. Clin. Chem. *23:* 2242-2246.

Schumann, G. B., and Greenberg, N. F. (1979). Usefulness of Macroscopic Urinalysis as a Screening Procedure. Am. J. Clin. Path., *71:* 425-426.

Smith, B. C., Peake, M. J. and Fraser, C. G. (1977). Urinalysis by Use of Multitest Reagent Strips. Two Dipsticks Compared. Clin. Chem., *23:* 2337-2340.

Stevens, J. B., and Osborne, C. A. (1974). Urinalysis: Indications, Methodology, and Interpretation. In: *Proc. 41st Annual AAHA Meeting.*

Sunderman, F. W., and Sunderman, F. W., Jr. (1970). *Laboratory Diagnosis of Kidney Diseases.* Publ. Warren H. Green, Inc., St. Louis, MO.

Thomas, G. H., and Howell, R. R. (1973). *Selected Screening Tests for Genetic Metabolic diseases.* Publ. Year Book Medical Publ., Chicago, IL.

Tietz, N. W. (1970). *Fundamentals of Clinical Chemistry.* Publ. W. B. Saunders Co., Philadelphia PA.

Wilkinson, J. W. (1969). Kidney Disease and Urine Analysis. In: *Textbook of Veterinary Clinical Pathology.* Medway, W. *et al.,* Ed. Publ. Williams & Wilkins Co., Baltimore, MD.

Osborne, C. A., Johnston, G. R., and Schenk, M. P. (1977). Cystocentesis: Indications, Contraindications, Technique, and Complications. Minn. Vet., *17:* 9-14.

Osborne, C. A., and Schenk, M. P. (1977). Techniques of Urine Collection. In: *Proc. 44th Annual AAHA Meeting.*

URINE OSMOLALITY, SPECIFIC GRAVITY, AND REFRACTIVE INDEX

Bovee, K. C. (1969). Urine Osmolality as a Definitive Indicator of Renal Concentrating Ability. JAVMA, *155:* 30-35.

Bovee, K. C. (1977).Diabetes insipidus, Vet. Clin. North Am., *7:* 603-611.

Feeney, D. A., Osborne, C. A., and Jessen, C. R. (1980). Effects of Radiographic Contrast Media on Results of Urinalysis with Emphasis on Alteration in specific Gravity. JAVMA, *176:* 1378-1381.

Green, R. A. (1978). Perspectives of Clinical Osmometry. Vet. Clin. North A., *8:* 287-299.

Greene, C. E., Wong, P. L., and Finco, D. R. (1979). Diagnosis and Treatment of Diabetes insipidus in Two Dogs Using Two Synthetic Analogs of Antidiuretic Hormone. JAAHA, *15:* 371-377.

Hardy, R. M., and Osborne, C. A. (1979). Water Deprivation Test in the Dog: Maximum Normal Values, JAVMA, *174:* 479-483.

Hays, R. M. (1976). Antidiuretic Hormone. NEJM, *295:* 659-665.

Jamison, R. L., and Maffly, R. H. (1976). The Urinary Concentrating Mechanism. NEJM, *295:* 1059-1076.

Lees, G. E. , Osborne, C. A., and Stevens, J. B. (1979). Antibacterial Properties or Urine: Studies of Feline specific Gravity, osmolality and pH. JAAHA, *15:* 135-141.

Madewell, B. R. Osborne, C. A., Norrdin, R. A., Stevens, J. B., and Hardy, R. M. (1975). Clinico-pathologic Aspects of diabetes insipidus in the Dog. JAAHA, *11:* 497-506.

O'Conner, W. J. and Potts, D. J. (1969). The External Water Exchanges of Normal Laboratory dogs. Quart. J. Exp. Physiol., *54:* 244-265.

Wolf, A. V., and Pillay, V. K. G. (1969). Renal Concentration Tests, Osmotic Pressure, Specific Gravity, and Electrical Conductivity Compared. Am. J. Med., *46:* 837-843.

Zwelling, L. A., and Balow, J. E. (1978). Hypersthenuria in High Dose Carbennicillin Therapy. Ann. Int. Med., *89:* 225-226.

URINE pH

Chow, F. H. C., Taton, G. F., Lewis, L. D., and Hamar, D. W. (1978). Effects of Dietary Ammonium Chloride, *dl*-Methionine, Sodium Phosphate and Ascorbic Acid on Urinary pH and Electrolyte Concentrations in Male Cats. Feline Pract., *8:* 29-34.

Lees, G. E., Osborne, C. A., and Stevens, J. B. (1979). Antibacterial Properties of Urine: Studies of Feline Specific Gravity, Osmolality and pH. JAAHA, *15:* 135-141.

Osborne, C.A., Stevens, J. B., Polzin, D. J., and Klausner, J. S. (1981). Clinical Significance of Urine pH. Minn. Vet., *21:* 24-27.

Brandt, R., Guyer, K. E., and Banks, W. L. (1977). Urinary Glucose and Vitamin C. Am. J. Clin. Path., *68:* 592-594.

Chinard, F. P., Taylor, W. R., Nolan, M. F., and Enns, T. (1959). Renal Handling of Glucose in Dogs. Am. J. Physiol., *196:* 535-544.

Free, A. H., and Free, H. M. (1975). Urine Sugar Testing—State of the Art. Lab. Med., *6:* 23-29.

Harrower, A. D. B., Campbell, I. W., Campbell, C. J., and McMaster, R. S. (1974). Diastix in the Estimation of Urinary Glucose. Practitioner, *213:* 241-245.

James, G. P., and Bee, D. E. (1979). Glucosuria: Accuracy and Precision of Laboratory Diagnosis by Dipstick Analysis. Clin. chem., *25:* 996-1001.

Keller, D. M. (1968). Glucose Excretion in Man and Dog. Nephron, *5:* 43-66.

MacCara, M. E., and Angaran, D. M. (1978). Cephalosporin—Clinitest Interaction: Comparison of Cephalothin, Am. J. Hosp. Pharm., *35:* 1064-1067.

Morrill, J., *et al.* (1974). Interference with Urinary Glucose determination by cephalothin. JAMA. *230:* 822-823.

Osborne, C. A., Stevens, J. M., Rakich, P., and Ogden, B. (1980). Clinical Significance of Glucosuria. Minn. Vet., *20:* 16-25.

Smith, D., and Young, W. W. (1977). Effect of Large Dose Ascorbic Acid on the Two-Drop Clinitest Determination. Am. J. Hosp. Pharm., *34:* 1347-1349.

Steirteghem, A. C., Robertson, E. A., and Young, D. S. (1978). Influence of Large Doses of Ascorbic Acid on Laboratory Test Results. Clin. Chem., *24:* 54-57.

Watts, C. (1968). Failure of Impregnated cellulose Strip as a Test for Glucose in Urine. Vet. Rec., *83:* 48-52.

PROTEINURIA

Alpert, H. C., Lohavichan, C., Presser, J. I., and Papper, S. (1974). Febrile Proteinuria. Southern Med. J., *67:* 552-554.

Aukland, K. (1960). Stop Flow Analysis of Renal Protein Excretion in the Dog. Scand. J. Lab. Invest., *12:* 300.

Barsanti, J. A., and Finco, D. R. (1979). Protein Concentration in Urine of Normal Dogs. AJVR, *40:* 1583-1588.

Brenner, B. M., Bohrer, M. P., Bayliss, C., and Deer, W. M. (1977). Determinants of Glomerular Permselectivity: Insights Derived from Observations *in vitro.* Kidney International, *12:* 229-237.

Carone, F. A., Peterson, D. R., Oparil, S., and Pullman, R. N. (1979). Renal Tubular Transport and Catabolism of Proteins and Peptides. Kidney International, *16:* 271-278.

DiBartola, S.P., Chew, D.J., and Jacobs, G. (1980). Quantitative Urinalysis Including 24-Hour Protein Excretion in the Dog. J. Am. Animal Hosp. Assoc., *16:* 537-546.

Dirks, J. H., Clapp, J. R., and Berliner, R. W. (1964). The Protein Concentration in the Proximal Tubles of the Dog. J. Clin. Invest., *43:* 916-921.

Gyure, W. L. (1977). Comparisons of Several Methods for Semiquantitative Determination of Urine Protein. Clin. Chem., *23:* 876-879.

Heinemann, H. D., Maack, T. M., and Sherman, R. L. (1974). Proteinuria. Am. J. Med., *56:* 71-82.

Hendriks, H. J., Hauge, A., and DeBuyne, J. J. (1976). Determination of the Protein Concentration in Canine Urine. Zbl. Vet. Med. A., *23:* 683-687.

Hurvitz, A. I., Kehoe, M., Capra, J. D., and Prata, R. (1971). Bence Jones Proteinemia and Proteinuria in the Dog. JAVMA, *159:* 1112-1116.

Osborne, C. A., and Stevens, J. B. (1978). Clinical Significance of Proteinuria. In: *Proc. 45th Annual AAHA Meeting.*

Pesce, A. J. (1974). Methods Used for the Analysis of Proteins in Urine. Nephron, *13:* 93-104.

Porter, P. (1964). Comparative Study of the Macromolecular Components Excreted in the Urine of Dog and Man. J. Comp. Path., *74:* 108-118.

Richardson, R. C. (1975). Interpretation of Urine Electrophoresis in Renal disease of the Canine. IN: *Proc. 42nd Annual AAHA Meeting.*

Stuart, B. P., Phemister, R. D., and Thomassen, R. W. (1975). Glomerular Lesions Associated with Proteinuria in clinically Healthy dogs. Vet. Pathol., *12:* 125-144.

Thysell, H. (1969). A Comparison between Albustix, Hemacombistix, Labstix, the Sulfosalicylic Acid Test, Heller's Nitric Acid Test, and a Biuret Method. Acta Med. Scand., *185:* 401-407.

OCCULT BLOOD, HEMOGLOBIN, AND MYOGLOBIN

Adams, E. C., and Rozman, M. J. (1970). Differentiation of Hemoglobinuria and Myoglobinuria in Renal Diseases In: *Laboratory Diagnosis of Kidney Diseases.* Sunderman, F. W., and Sunderman, F. W. Jr. (Ed). Publ. Warren H. Green, Inc., St. Louis, MO.

Boulton, F. E., and Huntsman, R. G. (1971). The Detection of Myoglobin in Urine and Its Distinction from Normal and Variant Hemoglobins. J. Clin. Path., *24:* 816-821.

Chu, S. Y., Curtis, C., and Turkington, V. E. (1978). Influence of pH on the Simple Solubility Test for Myoglobinuria. Clin. Biochem., *11:* 230-231.

Rowland, L. P., and Penn, A. S. (1972). Myoglobinuria. Med. Clin. North Am., *56:* 1233-1256.

BILIRUBIN

Cameron, J. L., Stafford, E. S., Schraufer, L., and Iber, F. L. (1963). Bilirubin Excretion in the Dog. J. Surg. Res., *3:* 39-42.

DeSchepper, J. (1974). Degradation of Hemoglobin to Bilirubin in the Kidney of the Dog. Tijdschr. Diergeneesk., *99:* 699-707.

DeSchepper, J. and VanDerStock, J. (1971). Influence of Sex on the Urinary Bilirubin Excretion at Increased Free Plasma Hemoglobin Levels in Whole Dogs and in Isolated Normothermic Perfused Dog Kidneys. Experentia, *27:* 1264-1265.

Fulop, M., and Brazeau, P. (1964). The Renal Excretion of Bilirubin in Dogs with Obstructive Jaundice. J. Clin. Invest., *43:* 1192-1202.

Fulop, M., and Brazeau, P. (1970). Impaired Renal Function Exaggerates Hyperbilirubinemia in Bile-Duct Ligated Dogs. Digestive Dis., *15:* 1067-1072.

Osborne, C. A., Stevens, J. B., Lees, G. E., Barlough, J. E., and Hardy, R. M. (1980). Clinical Significance of Bilirubinuria. Compend. on Cont. Educ. Small Anim. Prac., *2:* 897-902.

Schmid, R. (1972). Bilirubin Metabolism in Man. NEJM, *287:* 703-709.

UROBILINOGEN

Levy, M. Lester, R., and Levinsky, N. G. (1968). Renal Excretion of Urobilinogen in the Dog. J. Clin. Invest., *47:* 2117-2124.

URINE SEDIMENT

Alfthan, O. S., and Liewendahl, K. (1972). Investigation of Sulfonamide Crystalluria in Man. Scand. J. Urol., Nephrol., *6:* 44-46.

Bailey, D. N., and Jatlow, P. I. (1972). Chemical Analysis of Massive Crystalluria Following Primidone Overdose. Am. J. Clin. Path., *58:* 583-589.

Barlough, J.E., Osborne, C.A., and Stevens, J.B. (1980). Canine and Feline Urinalysis: Value of Macroscopic and Microscopic Examinations. JAVM, *178:* 611-63.

deVoogt, H. J., Rathert, P., and Beyer-Boon, M. E. (1977). *Urinary Cytology.* Publ. Springer-Verlag, New York, NY.

Gedcholt, H. (1968). Persistent of Blood Cells in Urine. Acta Med. Scand., *183:* 49-54

Glenn, B. L. (1970). Facts and Artifacts in the Microscopic Examination of Urine Sediment. JAVMA, *157:* 1667-1671.

Goulden, B. E. (1968). Assessment of the Usefulness of the Examination of a Gram Smear of Fresh Uncentrifuged Urine in the Determination of Significant Bacteriuria in Dogs. New Zealand Vet., J., *16:* 1.

Habner, M. H. (1972). Interference Contrast Microscopy for Identification of Urinary Sediments. Am. J. Clin. Path., *57:* 316-319.

Hindman, R., Tronic, B., and Bartlett, R. (1976). Effect of Delay on Urine Culture. J. Clin. Microbiol., *4:* 102-103.

Hoyer, J. R., and Seiler, M. W. (1979). Pathophysiology of Tamm-Horsfall Protein. Kidney International, *16:* 279-289.

Jones, H. M., and Schrader, W. A. (1972). Ampicillin Crystalluria. Am. J. Clin. Path., *58:* 220-223.

Lam, C. N. Bremmer, A. D., Maxwell, J. D., Murphy, A. V., and Low, W. J. (1967). Pyuria and Bacteriuria. Arch. Dis. Childh., *42:* 275-280.

Ling, G. V., and Kaneko, J. J. (1976). Microscopic Examination of Canine Urine Sediment. Calif. Vet., *30:* 14-18.

McIntyre, M., and Mou, T. W. (1965). Persistence of Leucocytes and Erythrocytes in Refrigerated and Alkaline Urine. Am. J. Clin. Path., *43:* 53-57.

McQueen, E. G. (1966). Composition of Urinary Casts. Lancet, *1:* 397.

Orita, Y., Imai, N. Ueda, N., Aoki, K., Sugimoto, K., Ando, A., Fujiwara, Y., Hirano, S., and Abe, H. (1977) Immunofluorescent Studies of Urinary Casts. Nephron, *19:* 19-25.

Osborne, C. A., and Stevens, J. B. (1978). *Digest of Canine and feline Urine Sediment.* Publ. Ralston Purina Co., St. Louis, MO.

Padilla, J., Osborne, C.A., and Ward, G.E. (1981). Effects of Storage Time and Temperature on Quantitative Urine Culture of Canine Urine. *178:* 1077-1081.

Prescott, L. F. (1966). The Normal Excretion Rates of Renal Tubular Cells, Leucocytes, and Red Blood Cells. Clin. Sci., *31:* 425-435.

Robertson, M. R., and Potter, E. (1973). The Significance of Plasma Proteins in Urinary Casts. Nephron, *11:* 294-307.

Rutecki, G. J., Goldsmith, C., and Schreiner, G. E. (1971). Characterization of Proteins in Urinary Casts. NEJM, *284:* 1049-1052.

Schumann, G. B., and Greenberg, N. F. (1978). Does Brightfield Microscopy Really Analyze Urine Sediment. Lab. Med., *9:* 23-26.

Schumann, G. B., Harris, S., and Henry, J. B. (1978). An Improved Technique for Examining Urinary Casts and a Review of Their Significance. Am. J. Clin. Path., *69:* 18-23.

Sternheimer, R. (1975). A Supravital Cytodiagnostic Stain for Urinary Sediment. JAMA, *231:* 826-832.

Stevens, J. B., and Osborne, C. A. (1978). Urinary Casts: What Are Their Significance. Minn. Vet., *18:* 11-18.

Vaughan, E. D., and Wyker, A. W. (1971). Effect of Osmolality on the Evaluation of Microscopic Hematuria. J. Urol., *105:* 709-711.

Winkel, P., Statland, B. E., and Jorgensen, K. (1974). Urine Microscopy, an Ill-defined Method, Examined by a Multifactorial Technique. Clin. Chem., *20:* 436-439.

Wise, G. J., Kozinn, P. J., and Toni, E. (1973). Yeast in the Urine. AFP, *7:* 120-125.

Wolfson, W. L., and Rosenthal, D. L. (1978). Cell Clusters in Urinary Cytology. Acta Cytologica, *22:* 138-141.

Sources of Supplies for Routine Urinalysis

Reagents– Diagnostic Strips

	Albustix®	Bili-Labstix®	Chemstrip® 3	Chemstrip® 4	Chemstrip® 5	Chemstrip® 6	Chemstrip® 7	Chemstrip® 8	Chemstrip® G	Chemstrip® GK	Clinistix® GP	Combistix®	C-Stix®	Diastix®	Hema-Combistix®	Hemastix®	Ictostix®	Keto-Diastix®	Ketostix®	Labstix®	Lo-Buff pHydrion®	Microstix®	Multistix®	Multistix® H	N-Multistix®	TesTape®	Urobilistix®	Uristix®
Ames Company Division of Miles Lab., Inc. P. O. Box 70 Elkhart, IN 46515	●	●									●	●	●	●	●	●	●	●	●	●		●	●	●	●		●	●
Bio-Dynamics 9115 Hague Road Indianapolis, IN 46206			●	●	●	●	●	●	●	●																		
Eli Lilly & Co. P. O. Box 1750 Indianapolis, IN 46206																										●		
Micro-Essential Laboratories 4224 Avenue North Brooklyn NY 11210																					●							

Reagents– Diagnostic Tablets/ Quality Control/ Stains

	Acetest®	Albustix®	Bumintest®	Clinitest®	Ictotest®	Hematest®	Kova-Trol®	Tek-Chek® 1	Tek-Chek® 2	Tek-Chek® 3	Tek-Chek® 4	Urintrol®	Gram Stain	New Methylene Blue Stain	Sedistain	Sudan III & IV	Wright's Stain
Ames Company Division of Miles Lab., Inc. P. O. Box 70 Elkhart, IN 46515	●	●	●	●	●	●	●	●	●	●							
Clay Adams Inc. Div. of Becton, Dickenon & Co. 299 Webro Road Parsippany, NJ 07054															●		
Fischer Scientific Co. 711 Forbes Avenue Pittsburgh, PA 15219													●	●			●
Harleco 60th & Woodland Avenue Philadelphia, PA 19104												●					
ICL Scientific 18249 Euclid St. Fountain Valley, CA 92708							●										
Matheson, Coleman and Bell Norwood, OH 45212													●			●	

Equipment & Suppliers

$\longrightarrow$

Equipment & Suppliers

	ANESTHETICS	AUTOCLAVES	CANNULAS		CATHETERS					
					Human		Canine		Feline	
	Anestacon®	Sterilizer	Silver Abscess	Ureteral	Uretheral (Foley)	Flexible plastic	Flexible rubber	Swan Ganz Flow Balloon	Infant feeding Tubes	Jackson cat
American Cystoscope Makers Inc. 8 Pelham Parkway Pelham Manor, NY 10803				●						
American Hospital Supply Co. Scientific Products Division 1430 Waukegan Road, McGaw Park, IL 60085		●								
American Optical Scientific Instrument Division P. O. Box 123, Buffalo, NY 14215										
C. R. Bard, Inc. Bard Hospital Division Murray Hill, NJ 07974				●	●					
Becton-Dickenson & Company Rutherford, NJ 07974			●							
Clay Adams Inc. Div. of Becton, Dickenson & Co. 299 Webro Road, Parsippany, NJ 07054										
Conal Pharmaceuticals Inc. Chicago, IL 60640	●									
Cutter Laboratories Inc. Berkeley, CA 94710				●	●					
Edwards Laboratories 17221 Red Hill Avenue Santa Ana, CA 92705								●		
Fisher Scientific Company 711 Forbes Avenue Pittsburgh, Pennsylvania 15219		●								
Haver Lockhart Labs. Box 390 Shawnee, KS 66201						●				
Life-Tech Instruments Inc. Box 36221 Houston, TX 77036				●	●					
Med-Tech Inc. P. O. Box 338 Elwood, KS 66024										
V. Mueller Co. Chicago, IL		●								
Pharmaseal Inc. Toa Alta, Puerto Rico 00758										
Phylab Division Physicians Hosp. & Sply Co. Minneapolis, MN 55403										
Portex Wilmington, MA 01887										●
Sherwood Medical Industries Inc. 1831 Olive Street St. Louis, MO 63103						●	●		●	
Welch-Allyn, Inc. Shaneateles Falls, NY 13153										

Index

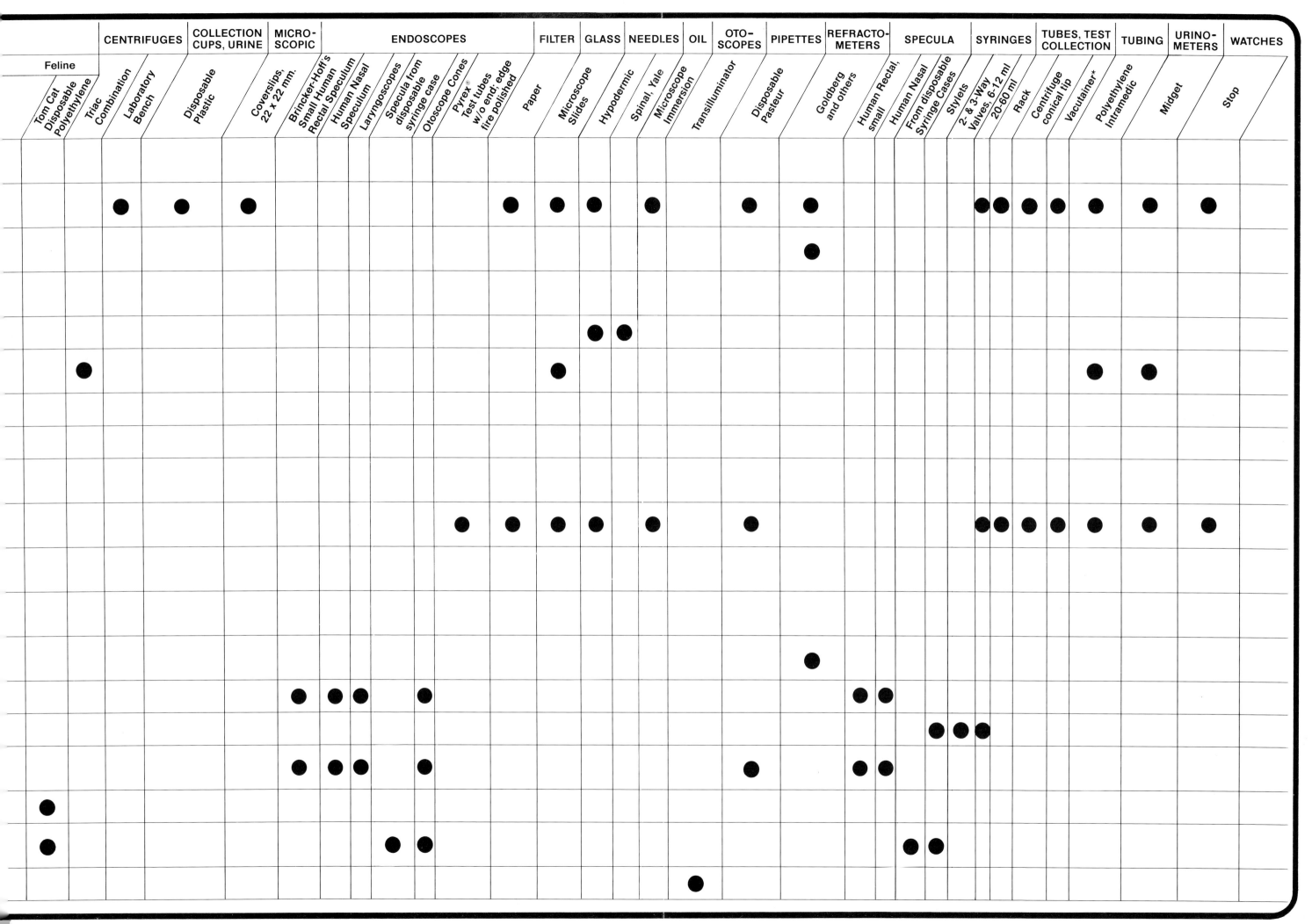